Handbook on
Epilepsy for Physicians

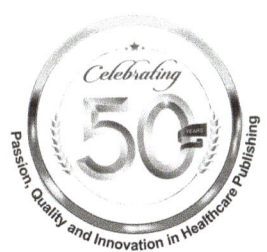

In pursuit of good care of people with Epilepsy

With Compliments from:
Indian Epilepsy Association Bangalore Chapter

Handbook on
Epilepsy for Physicians

Editors

PV Rai
Senior Neurologist/Epileptologist
Former Associate Medical Director
Swiss Epilepsy Center
Zurich, Switzerland

HV Srinivas
Senior Consultant
Neurologist, Sagar Hospital and
Agadi Hospital, Bengaluru
Former Associate Professor
Department of Neurology
NIMHANS, Bengaluru, Karnataka, India

P Satishchandra
Advisor and Senior Consultant
Department of Neurology/Epileptology
Apollo Hospitals, Bengaluru
Hon. Professor
University of Liverpool, UK
Former Director
Vice-Chancellor and
Ex-Senior Professor
Department of Neurology
National Institute of Mental Health and
Neurosciences (NIMHANS)
Bengaluru, Karnataka, India

GT Subhas
Senior Consultant
Neurologist/Epileptologist
Former Dean/Director
Bangalore Medical College and
Research Institute
Professor and Head
Department of Neurology
BMCRI, Bengaluru, Karnataka, India

Foreword
Bhim S Singhal

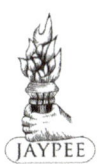

JAYPEE BROTHERS MEDICAL PUBLISHERS
The Health Sciences Publisher
New Delhi | London | Panama

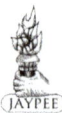 **Jaypee Brothers Medical Publishers (P) Ltd**

Headquarters
Jaypee Brothers Medical Publishers (P) Ltd
4838/24, Ansari Road, Daryaganj
New Delhi 110 002, India
Phone: +91-11-43574357
Fax: +91-11-43574314
E-mail: jaypee@jaypeebrothers.com

Overseas Offices
JP Medical Ltd
83 Victoria Street, London
SW1H 0HW (UK)
Phone: +44 20 3170 8910
Fax: +44 (0)20 3008 6180
E-mail: info@jpmedpub.com

Jaypee-Highlights Medical Publishers Inc
City of Knowledge, Bld. 235, 2nd Floor, Clayton
Panama City, Panama
Phone: +1 507-301-0496
Fax: +1 507-301-0499
E-mail: cservice@jphmedical.com

Jaypee Brothers Medical Publishers (P) Ltd
Bhotahity, Kathmandu, Nepal
Phone: +977-9741283608
E-mail: kathmandu@jaypeebrothers.com

Website: www.jaypeebrothers.com
Website: www.jaypeedigital.com

© 2019, Jaypee Brothers Medical Publishers

The views and opinions expressed in this book are solely those of the original contributor(s)/author(s) and do not necessarily represent those of editor(s) of the book.

All rights reserved. No part of this publication may be reproduced, stored or transmitted in any form or by any means, electronic, mechanical, photocopying, recording or otherwise, without the prior permission in writing of the publishers.

All brand names and product names used in this book are trade names, service marks, trademarks or registered trademarks of their respective owners. The publisher is not associated with any product or vendor mentioned in this book.

Medical knowledge and practice change constantly. This book is designed to provide accurate, authoritative information about the subject matter in question. However, readers are advised to check the most current information available on procedures included and check information from the manufacturer of each product to be administered, to verify the recommended dose, formula, method and duration of administration, adverse effects and contraindications. It is the responsibility of the practitioner to take all appropriate safety precautions. Neither the publisher nor the author(s)/editor(s) assume any liability for any injury and/or damage to persons or property arising from or related to use of material in this book.

This book is sold on the understanding that the publisher is not engaged in providing professional medical services. If such advice or services are required, the services of a competent medical professional should be sought.

Every effort has been made where necessary to contact holders of copyright to obtain permission to reproduce copyright material. If any have been inadvertently overlooked, the publisher will be pleased to make the necessary arrangements at the first opportunity. The **CD/DVD-ROM** (if any) provided in the sealed envelope with this book is complimentary and free of cost. **Not meant for sale.**

Inquiries for bulk sales may be solicited at: jaypee@jaypeebrothers.com

Handbook on Epilepsy for Physicians

First Edition: 2019

ISBN: 978-93-89188-00-4

Dedicated to

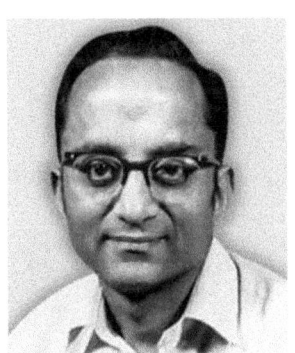

Late Dr KS Mani

*Founder Member of Indian Epilepsy Association
National Body and Bangalore Chapter
"Father of Indian Epileptology"*

Contributors

Agadi JB
Senior Consultant Neurologist
Apollo Hospitals, Bengaluru
Former Professor and Head
Department of Neurology
Bangalore Medical College and
Research Institute
Bengaluru, Karnataka, India

Akshita Hariharan
MPhil in Clinical Psychology
Clinical Neuropsychologist
Consultant at Agadi Hospital and
Vikram Hospital
Bengaluru, Karnataka, India

Bhaskara Rao Malla
Professor and Head
Department of Neurosurgery
National Institute of Mental Health and
Neurosciences
Bengaluru, Karnataka, India

Chanda Kulkarni
Advisor—Clinical Pharmacology
Sakra World Hospital
Bengaluru, Karnataka, India

Damodar Rao HK
Hon. Secretary
Indian Epilepsy Association
Bangalore Chapter
Bengaluru, Karnataka, India

Delon D'Souza
Assistant Professor
Department of Neurology
St John's Medical College and Hospital
Bengaluru, Karnataka, India

Inbaraj G
PhD Scholar
Department of Neurophysiology
National Institute of Mental Health and
Neurosciences
Bengaluru, Karnataka, India

Johnson Pradeep R
Associate Professor
Psychiatry, Medical Ethics
Institutional Ethics Committee (IEC)
St John's Medical College and Hospital
Bengaluru, Karnataka, India

Kalyanasundaram S
Consultant Psychiatrist and
Hon. Secretary
The Richmond Fellowship Society (India)
Bengaluru, Karnataka, India

Muralidharan KV
Hon. Treasurer, Indian Epilepsy
Association, Central Office
Epilepsy Counselor, Indian Epilepsy
Association, Bangalore Chapter
Bengaluru, Karnataka, India

Priyamvada Tatachar
Attending Epileptologist
Ann and Robert H Lurie
Children's Hospital
Assistant Professor
Department of Pediatrics and Neurology
Northwestern University
Feinberg School of Medicine
Chicago, Illinois, USA

Raghavendra K
Assistant Professor
Department of Neurology
National Institute of Mental Health and
Neurosciences
Bengaluru, Karnataka, India

Rai PV
Senior Neurologist/Epileptologist
Former Associate Medical Director
Swiss Epilepsy Center
Zurich, Switzerland

Rajendra P Joshi
Senior Chief Medical Officer (SAG)
Central Health Services
Bengaluru, Karnataka, India

Ravindranadh Chowdary M
Associate Professor
Department of Neurology
National Institute of Mental Health and
Neurosciences
Bengaluru, Karnataka, India

Sanjib Sinha
Professor and Head
Department of Neurology
National Institute of Mental Health and
Neurosciences
Bengaluru, Karnataka, India

Sarma GRK
Professor
Department of Neurology
St Johns Medical College
Bengaluru, Karnataka, India

Sathyaprabha TN
Professor and Head
Department of Neurophysiology
National Institute of Mental Health and
Neurosciences
Bengaluru, Karnataka, India

Satishchandra P
Advisor and Senior Consultant
Department of Neurology/Epileptology
Apollo Hospitals, Bengaluru
Former Director, Vice-Chancellor and
Ex-Senior Professor
Department of Neurology
National Institute of Mental Health and
Neurosciences
Bengaluru, Karnataka, India

Shishir Duble
Assistant Professor (Ad-hoc)
Department of Neurology
National Institute of Mental Health and
Neurosciences
Bengaluru, Karnataka, India

Shiva Kumar R
Senior Consultant Epileptologist and
Neurologist
Institute of Neurosciences
Sakra World Hospital
Bengaluru, Karnataka, India

Sreeram AC
Senior Consultant Physician
Director, Mallige Hospital
Bengaluru, Karnataka, India

Srinivas HV
Senior Consultant Neurologist
Sagar Hospital and Agadi Hospital
Bengaluru, Karnataka, India

Subhas GT
Former Dean/Director
Bangalore Medical College and
Research Institute (BMCRI)
Professor and Head
Department of Neurology
BMCRI (1996–2013)
Bengaluru, Karnataka, India

Sujit Kumar
Consultant Neurologist and Epileptologist
Apollo Hospitals
Bengaluru, Karnataka, India

Thomas Mathew
Professor and Head
Department of Neurology
St John's Medical College and Hospital
Bengaluru, Karnataka, India

Viswanathan LG
Postdoctoral Fellow (Epilepsy)
National Institute of Mental Health and
Neurosciences
Bengaluru, Karnataka, India

Foreword

I am honored to write the foreword for the book *"Handbook on Epilepsy for Physicians",* brought out by Indian Epilepsy Association (IEA) Bangalore Chapter. Epilepsy is a common neurological problem seen in day-to-day practice of primary care physicians. Epilepsy can be diagnosed clinically and managed easily in about 70–80% of patients. However, due to paucity of adequate training and knowledge, this eminently treatable condition is often misdiagnosed and not managed correctly. This book addresses several such issues and is handy for the Physicians to quickly refer and make a proper diagnosis and manage.

I should compliment the four distinguished editors for this multi-authored book. They have invited specialists with expertise in the field of epilepsy and having a large practical experience in managing persons with epilepsy to write the various chapters. Each section is devoted to one aspect of epilepsy, which includes diagnosis, investigations, and appropriate management.

The book also dwells into difficult to treat epilepsy/drug-resistant epilepsy, which accounts for about 20–25% of all epilepsies. Investigation of such a case along with the indications for surgery has been well brought out. For readers who would like to have some advanced information, the role of genetics and personalized treatment has been touched upon.

Indian Epilepsy Association Bangalore Chapter has been in the forefront of public education to dispel the myths and misunderstanding about epilepsy. For more than 10 years, members of the Association have been addressing regularly students in schools, colleges, and various social organizations. In addition, street plays are being performed regularly for more than 10 years, by amateur artists to spread the right message to rural and semiurban population. These are conducted in busy places such as bus stand, railway station, schools, and weekly fairs. It is heartening to note that the book also covers several social aspects of epilepsy, which the medical doctors should be aware of to educate their patients and their family members.

This comprehensive *"Handbook on Epilepsy for Physicians"* should be extremely useful for all those who care for persons with epilepsy including family physicians, internists, pediatricians, neurologists, and psychiatrists.

Bhim S Singhal
Director of Neurology
Bombay Hospital Institute of Medical Sciences
Mumbai, Maharashtra, India

Preface

For the past four to five decades, there has been significant advancement in the diagnosis and treatment for people living with epilepsy (PWE). This is the result of some major developments in the field of neurology and neurosciences, which have resulted in the establishment of a specialization—Epileptology. The progress in epileptology can be traced mainly to three to four major areas such as: (1) the classification of epileptic seizures and epilepsies—by the International League against Epilepsy (ILAE), (2) the development of newer antiepileptic drugs (AEDs), (3) the advancement in the field of medical technology—in particular electroencephalography (EEG) with different forms of application—neuroradiological investigations with computed tomography (CT) scan, magnetic resonance imaging (MRI), positron emission tomography (PET), etc. Further progress is the result of extensive scientific and social programs carried out by the two organizations—ILAE and International Bureau for Epilepsy (IBE) through their worldwide chapters.

Because of these advancements, epilepsy, which was for ages considered as "incurable", has become an eminently treatable neurological condition with over 70% PWE almost certain to achieve the status of freedom from seizures. Having a variety AEDs available in the market, with proper selection, a single drug can lead to seizure freedom in about 70%. Where drugs do not help, in a small number of people, neurosurgery can make a person free of seizures. Under this positive scenario of epilepsy treatment, the reality is very much different particularly in developing countries including India. A large number of PWE mostly in the rural areas do not get even the basic drug treatment and continue to have seizures, although some of the effective "standard" drugs have become cost-effective and affordable for all sections of society.

Epilepsy is very much a clinical condition. The diagnosis of epilepsy is made on the basis of identification of seizures and the circumstances, which lead to their manifestation. With ongoing Continuing Medical Education (CME) program around the year, every physician should be able to diagnose and treat a PWE in nearly 70% of cases, except in cases of some complicated epilepsies, where neurological consultation may be needed. Managing a PWE at the level of primary healthcare/general medical practice is of utmost importance in view of the present medical and social situation in India. The number of neurologists available in the country is insufficient for the management of huge population of around 10-12 million of PWE in India.

With this in our mind, the Indian Epilepsy Association (IEA) Bangalore Chapter has planned to have simple but comprehensive *"Handbook on Epilepsy for Physicians"*. We hope that this will guide our physicians in day-to-day practice in managing their patients. This is a multi-author book and the authors chosen for this task are highly proficient in their field of work related to epileptology. Thanks to their contribution, the book provides expert and latest information regarding various aspects of epilepsy.

Attempts have been made to present important aspects of epilepsy as separate chapters, so that the readers can select these chapters according to their particular needs. Examples, febrile seizures, new onset epilepsy, epilepsy syndromes in children, epilepsy in the elderly, seizures but not epilepsy, epilepsy and pregnancy, to name only a few of the chapters. The authors have done commendable work in synthesizing their ideas, taking much time, in spite of their busy professional schedule for which we express our gratitude to them.

The book would not have seen the light of the day at this stage of publication but for the incessant work of Dr HV Srinivas in doing maximum amount of the editorial work, in spite of his busy professional activity. He has dedicated weeks and months of his private time for bringing out a neurological book on epilepsy for physicians. We express our sincere thank profusely.

We wish to dedicate this book to our Indian Epilepsy Association founder Professor KS Mani who is known as "Father of Indian Epileptology". We are thankful to Professor BS Singhal for kindly writing the Foreword for this book. We also thank the Jaypee Brothers Medical Publishers (P) Ltd., New Delhi and their Bengaluru office for bringing out the book in a beautiful form.

Rai PV
Srinivas HV
Satishchandra P
Subhas GT

Acknowledgements

The book is a brainchild of Dr PV Rai, President of Indian Epilepsy Association Bangalore Chapter, who mooted the idea of bring out multi-authored book on behalf of Indian Epilepsy Association (IEA) Bangalore Chapter, which would be of help to Primary Care Physicians dealing with epilepsy.

Sincere thanks to all the contributors from IEA Bangalore Chapter who spared their time willingly to contribute to this book.

Our thanks to Dr BS Singhal for graciously accepting to write the Foreword.

The Editors wish to express their hearty thanks to Dr HV Srinivas for his untiring work of editing, organizing, and "endless" correspondence with Authors and Publishers.

We thank Ms Meena Chandramohan for diligently copyediting the book.

We thank our Secretary Ms Theresa Pinto for typing several drafts ungrudgingly before it took the final shape.

Finally, we are thankful to Shri Jitendar P Vij (Group Chairman), Mr Ankit Vij (Managing Director), Mr MS Mani (Group President), Ms Chetna Malhotra Vohra (Associate Director—Content Strategy), Ms Pooja Bhandari (Production Head) and Ms Nedup Denka Bhutia (Development Editor) of M/s Jaypee Brothers Medical Publishers (P) Ltd, New Delhi, India, for giving a go-ahead at the very beginning and helping us in every way possible to bring out this book.

Contents

1. **Short History of Epilepsy** 1
   Rai PV, Sreeram AC
   - Further Progress in Epilepsy Management *4*
   - Indian Scenario *6*

2. **Febrile Seizures** 7
   Subhas GT, Priyamvada Tatachar
   - Definition of Febrile Seizures *7*
   - Epidemiology: Burden of Problems *7*
   - Etiology: Predisposing Factors—Age *7*
   - Fever—Infections *8*
   - Immunization *8*
   - Genetics *8*
   - Other Associated Factors *8*
   - Clinical Features *9*
   - Classifications *9*
   - Diagnostic Evaluation *10*
   - Differential Diagnosis *10*
   - Treatment of Febrile Seizures in Its Acute Phase *11*
   - Recurrence Risk *12*
   - Prophylaxis *13*
   - Prognosis *14*
   - Parental Counseling *14*

3. **Epilepsy and Epilepsy Syndromes in Children** 16
   Raghavendra K
   - Epidemiology *16*
   - Approach to Child with Seizure *17*
   - Etiology *19*
   - Special Conditions in Children *23*
   - Comorbidity of Childhood Epilepsy *25*
   - Management *26*
   - Pediatric Intractable Epilepsy Syndromes *27*

4. **New-onset Epilepsy in Adults** 30
   Delon D'Souza, Thomas Mathew
   - Primary New-onset Epilepsy in Adults *31*
   - Secondary New-onset Epilepsy in Adults *34*
   - Investigations *38*

5. **Epilepsy in Elderly** 41
   Satishchandra P, Viswanathan LG, Sanjib Sinha
   - Epidemiology, Classification, and Etiology *42*
   - Provoked Seizures *42*
   - First Unprovoked Seizure and Epilepsy *43*
   - Diagnostic Evaluation *43*
   - Antiepileptic Drug Selection *44*
   - Antiepileptic Medications *44*
   - Status Epilepticus among Elderly *45*

6. **Women, Epilepsy and Pregnancy** 48
   Agadi JB
   - Effect of Pregnancy on Epilepsy *48*
   - Effect of Epilepsy on Pregnancy *48*
   - Teratogenic Effects of Antiepileptic Drugs *49*
   - Cognitive Teratogenesis *50*
   - Management Strategies *50*
   - Contraception *51*
   - Catamenial Epilepsy *52*

7. **Seizures but Not Epilepsy** 54
   Srinivas HV
   - Is it a Seizure? *54*
   - Is the Seizure Provoked? *55*
   - A Single Unprovoked Genuine Seizure—is it Epilepsy? *56*

8. **Epilepsy and Psychiatric Aspects** 58
   Kalyanasundaram S, Johnson Pradeep R
   Depression and Anxiety Disorders in People with Epilepsy 58
   - Epidemiology *58*
   - Clinical Features *59*
   - Etiologies *59*
   - Role of Antiepileptic Drugs *60*
   - Screening for Depression *60*
   - Treatment Strategies for Depression and Anxiety Disorders in Epilepsy *60*

Psychosis in Persons with Epilepsy   *61*
- Epidemiology   *61*
- Management   *64*

Personality in Persons with Epilepsy   *64*
- Temporal Lobe Epilepsy   *64*
- Juvenile Myoclonic Epilepsy   *64*
- Absence Epilepsy   *65*
- Frontal Lobe Epilepsy   *65*

9. **Genetics of Epilepsy** 67
   Shishir Duble, Sanjib Sinha, Satishchandra P
   - Genetic Basis of Epilepsy   *67*
   - Mendelian and Nonmendelian Inheritance   *69*
   - Epilepsy with Complex Inheritance or Nonmendelian   *69*
   - Mitochondrial Inheritance   *69*
   - Epigenetics   *71*
   - Pharmacogenetics of Epilepsy   *73*
   - Challenges in Genetic Testing   *74*

10. **Investigations in Epilepsy** 77
    Viswanathan LG, Satishchandra P, Sanjib Sinha
    - Electroencephalography   *77*
    - Other Electrophysiological Procedures   *80*
    - Imaging Modalities   *80*
    - Other Investigations for Epilepsy   *83*

11. **Emergencies in Epilepsy: Diagnosis and Management** 88
    Shiva Kumar R
    - Cluster Seizures (Acute Repetitive Seizures)   *88*
    - Status Epilepticus   *89*
    - Nonconvulsive Status Epilepticus   *96*

12. **Drug Treatment: Choice of Antiepileptic Drugs** 99
    Sujit Kumar
    - Goals of Treatment   *99*

13. **Diagnosis of Epilepsy** 107
    Sarma GRK
    - Level 1: Identification of Seizure Type   *107*
    - Level 2: Identification of Epilepsy Type   *109*
    - Level 3: Identification of Epilepsy Syndrome   *110*

- Etiology *111*
- Comorbidities *111*
- Investigation of Epilepsy *112*

14. Drug Withdrawal after Seizure Freedom: When and How? 115
Rai PV
- Benefits of Drug Withdrawal *116*
- Risks of Drug Withdrawal *117*
- Conditions Favorable for Drug Withdrawal *117*
- Conditions Unfavorable for Drug Withdrawal *118*
- Prognosis after Drug Withdrawal *118*
- Practical Guidelines for Drug Withdrawal *118*

15. Therapy Resistance and Management 122
Ravindranadh Chowdary M
- Definition and Its Evaluation *122*
- Epidemiology *122*
- Etiopathogenesis and Predictors of Refractory Epilepsy *122*
- Consequences of Refractory Epilepsy *123*
- Management *123*

16. Surgery for Epilepsy 129
Bhaskara Rao Malla
- Goal of Surgery *129*
- Surgically Remediable Syndromes *129*
- Presurgical Evaluation *130*
- Surgical Procedures *131*
- Contraindications *135*
- Outcomes *135*

17. Epilepsy and Counseling 137
Akshita Hariharan
- Impact of Diagnosis *137*
- Stigma *137*
- Counseling *138*
- Role of a Clinical Psychologist *141*

18. Prevention of Epilepsy 143
Chanda Kulkarni
- Primary Prevention *143*
- Secondary Prevention *144*

19. **Epilepsy and Law** 146
   Srinivas HV
   - Epilepsy and Marriage   *146*
   - Epilepsy and Driving   *146*
   - Epilepsy and Employment   *147*
   - Epilepsy and Disability   *147*
   - Epilepsy and Insurance   *147*
   - Epilepsy and Income Tax   *147*

20. **Epilepsy: Education and Employment** 148
   Rajendra P Joshi

21. **Role of Yoga, Exercise, and Leisure Activities in Patients with Epilepsy** 151
   Inbaraj G, Sathyaprabha TN
   - Epilepsy and Yoga   *151*
   - Epilepsy and Exercise   *152*
   - Epilepsy and Cognition   *153*

22. **Diet, Television and Computer** 156
   Damodar Rao HK

23. **Indian Epilepsy Association: A Brief History** 158
   Muralidharan KV
   - International Scenario   *158*
   - Birth of Indian Epilepsy Association   *159*
   - Activities of Indian Epilepsy Association   *160*
   - Annual Conferences   *160*
   - Indian Epilepsy Association: Bangalore Chapter   *160*

Appendices 163

Index 167

1

Short History of Epilepsy

Rai PV, Sreeram AC

INTRODUCTION

The history of epilepsy can be traced to early civilizations. The oldest mention is found in the Babylonian clay tablet, written in Sumerian language, during the reign of the Babylonian King Adad-apla-iddina (1067–1046 BC). The tablet, which is kept in the British Museum, is called "antashubba" meaning "falling disease" in Sumerian. This forms a part of such tablets on human diseases. Mention of epilepsy is found in the Bible, where Jesus Christ heals a boy with epilepsy. People then believed that epilepsy was caused by supernatural powers such as by Gods and evil spirits and the treatment consisted of driving away such spirits.

Ayurveda refers to epilepsy in the Charaka Samhita (1000–500 BC) as "Apasmara" and mentions several kinds of seizures, which are comparable to the present day clinical description. The cause of epilepsy is traced to the vitiation of three basic factors "Vata, Pitta, and Kapha" and the treatment consists in correction of these "Doshas". Hippocrates of Kos (460–370 BC) referred to as the "Father of Medicine" made major contributions for understanding of epilepsy. At his time, epilepsy was considered a "sacred disease" probably because famous people like Alexander the Great and Julius Caesar had this disease in spite of their great military and leadership qualities. Hippocrates, in his treatise on "Sacred Disease", declared epilepsy as a natural disease and traced its origin to the brain. He mentioned "it is thus with regard to the disease called sacred. It appears to me to be nowise more divine nor more sacred than other diseases, but has a natural cause from the originates like other affections. Men regard its nature and cause as divine from ignorance and wonder because it is not at all like other diseases. And, this notion of its divinity is kept up by their inability to comprehend it".[1]

Hippocrates examined the skulls of people with epilepsy (PWE), which had holes in them probably to drive away the evil spirits. After examining the brains of such people, he came to the conclusion that the brain must be the organ responsible for seizures. However, Hippocrates believed that the disturbance of bodily (and brain) humors was responsible for causing seizures and the treatment he suggested was correction of this humoral imbalance.

Several centuries after Hippocrates, the Greek Physician Claudius Galen (130-210 AD), who founded his school in Rome, accepted the Hippocratic concept of brain as the seat of epilepsy. Galen's theory on pathophysiology of diseases including epilepsy rested on the basis of bodily humors and the treatment consisted of their correction with diet, bloodletting, and other procedures. Galen classified epilepsy as "idiopathic" meaning caused by brain humors and "sympathetic" referring to other irritating factors. Both the schools of Hippocrates and Galen considered epilepsy as a major disease and called it "morbus sacer" and "morbus divus". The influence of these schools of ancient Greek medicine lasted for several generations but lost their significance over the succeeding centuries probably because of the lack of treatment against epileptic seizures. For centuries, PWE were at the mercy of faith healers and sorcerers of various kinds. Probably because of this situation, there is practically no mention on epilepsy in the history of medicine for the next 1,500 years.[2]

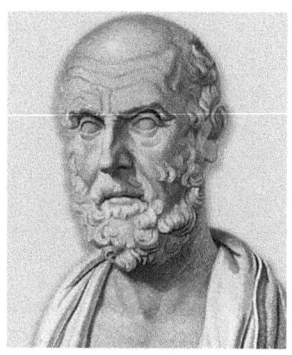

Hippocrates

The modern history of epilepsy can be traced to the early 19th century in West European countries, which more or less coincided with the Industrial Revolution and then spread rapidly to North America and other countries. A French Physician, Dominique Esquirol (1772-1840), classified epilepsy into "grand mal and petit mal" and differentiated epilepsy from psychiatric conditions. Two British neurologists, William Richard Gowers (1845-1915) and John Hughlings Jackson (1835-1911), made significant contributions toward understanding epilepsy as a functional disorder of the cerebral cortex. Around the first part of 19th century, neurology evolved itself into a separate medical discipline, away from psychiatry and internal medicine, depending upon the situation of the medical practice.

The clinical and scientific work of John Hughlings Jackson paved the way for the understanding of seizures as excessive neuronal discharge of brain hemisphere corresponding to the contralateral extremities, also in the form of "March of spasm". His work on the "Study of Convulsions" was a pathbreaker in the direction of "Epileptology" becoming a subspecialty of neurology.

Jackson devoted a major part of his professional career of over 40 years for the study of epilepsy, which formed the basis for further studies by his contemporaries and neurologists

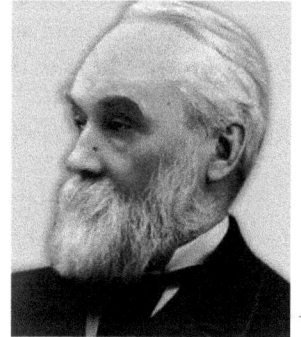

John Hughlings Jackson

of succeeding generations of 19th and 20th centuries. His definition that "epilepsy is the name for occasional, sudden, excessive, rapid, and local discharges of gray matter" holds good, particularly for focal epilepsies even today.[3] The beginning of the 20th century noticed further publications related to epilepsy from several distinguished neurologists.

William Richard Gowers published in 1881 a monograph "epilepsy and other chronic convulsive diseases". In 1907, he published his second book "The Borderland of Epilepsy" in which he referred to the differential diagnosis of other seizure-like conditions such as vertigo, vasovagal attacks, migraine, and narcolepsy. Gowers was known for his clinical accuracy and pathophysiology of epilepsy. His concept of "seizures beget seizures" has some clinical significance even today.

In 1924, Hans Berger (1873-1941), a German psychiatrist from the University of Jena, succeeded in recording the first human electroencephalogram (EEG), with which he had hoped to detect "the correlation between objective activity of the brain and subjective psychic phenomenon". After initial disappointment, he published his paper "recording the electrical activity of the human brain from the surface of the head" in 1929.[2]

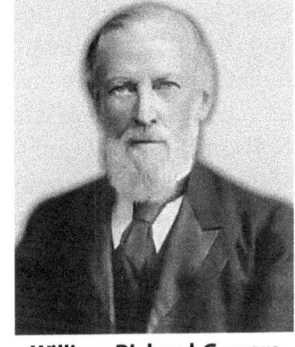
William Richard Gowers

The medical profession, to begin with, was somewhat skeptical of Berger's invention, but after it was certified by American and British neurophysiologists, EEG was technically improved and fully accepted as the method of investigation in the diagnosis/differential diagnosis of epilepsy, which continues even today, however, in a much sophisticated form.

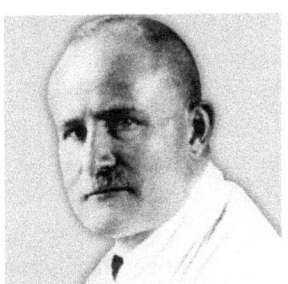
Hans Berger

William Gordon Lennox (1884-1960) was an American neurologist and a leading personality in the further development of Epileptology. He is widely known because of his intensive clinical and EEG work on childhood encephalopathy known as "Lennox-Gastaut syndrome" described later by another pioneer Henri Gastaut. Lennox developed interest for epilepsy during his service as a missionary Doctor in China and after returning to USA, he intensified his work on the severe form of childhood epilepsy syndrome making widespread EEG studies along with his colleagues Stanley Cobb, Erna, and Frederic Gibbs. His book "Epilepsy and

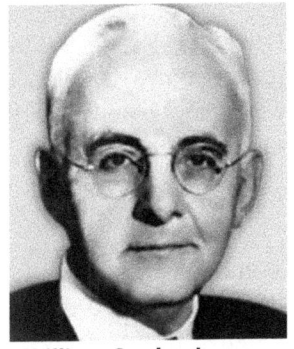
William Gordon Lennox

Related Disorders", co-authored with his daughter Margaret Buchtal, is popular even today. Lennox took active interest in the medicosocial aspects of epilepsy. He was president of the International League against Epilepsy (ILAE) from 1935 to 1946 and editor of the Journal Epilepsia from 1945 to 1950.[3]

Wilder Graves Penfield (1891-1976) was a famous Canadian neurosurgeon with multi-sided interest involving medicine, philosophy, and literature. In Epileptology, he is known for his pathbreaking work for surgically removing "epileptic neurons" where the seizures originate. Penfield operated patients on local anesthesia and before the operation he electrically stimulated the brain to observe the focus of origin of seizures in conscious patients. Along with Herbert Jasper, he published his leading book "Epilepsy and the Functional Anatomy of the Human Brain". Penfield's work has provided considerable service for the succeeding generation of neurosurgeons, neurologists, and epileptologists. Penfield has published several books on neuroanatomy, neurosurgery, epilepsy, psychology, and philosophy.[4]

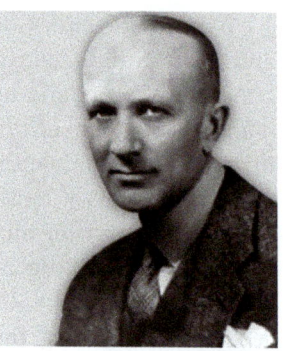

Wilder Graves Penfield

Henri Jean Pascal Gastaut (1915-1995) was a French neurologist who devoted his professional career in the service of Epileptology. He is widely known for the presentation of the Lennox-Gastaut syndrome, which he wished to publish in the name of William Lennox only, but the ILAE considering the efforts of Gastaut named the syndrome Lennox-Gastaut syndrome, under the initiative of Lennox's daughter Margaret Buchtal. Gastaut was actively involved in the activities of ILAE. He was the secretary general (1957-1969) and president (1969-1973) of ILAE. Gastaut is also known for the early classification of epileptic seizures and epilepsies by the ILAE, which has helped considerably in the clinical and EEG diagnosis/differential diagnosis of epilepsy.

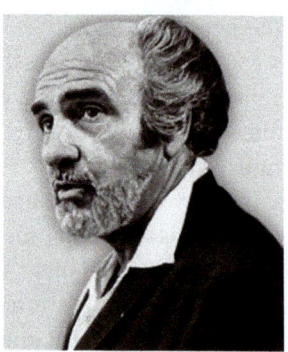

Henri Jean Pascal Gastaut

FURTHER PROGRESS IN EPILEPSY MANAGEMENT

A milestone in the history of epilepsy is the introduction of bromide, the first ever effective antiepileptic drug by Charles Locock in 1857. Although a sedative, it was widely used for around half a century in European countries and North America. In the mid-19th century, several homes and colonies for PWE were founded in West European countries mostly by the Christian missionaries. Examples of such centers are Bethel, Bielefeld in Germany, Heemstede in Netherlands, Chalfont Center in England, Swiss Epilepsy Center, Zurich, Switzerland, Epilepsy Center Dianalund in Denmark, and Epilepsy Center in Sandvika Norway. These centers over the next 100 years have developed into full-fledged epilepsy (neuro) centers, taking care of the medical and social needs of PWE.[5]

Another important development was the foundation of the ILAE as early as in 1909, with the initiative of eminent neurologists like John Hughlings Jackson. The goal of ILAE is to promote worldwide research in the field of epilepsy for improving the lives of PWE. ILAE gives frequent guidelines for medical professionals like offering International Classification of epileptic seizures and epilepsies. It also runs the medical journal "Epilepsia", which updates on epilepsy research and management. Much later in 1961, a second important organization, the International Bureau for Epilepsy (IBE), was founded by the initiatives of people like George Burden for the purpose of coordinating the social needs of PWE—on a worldwide basis. IBE has in its membership both medical professionals and the general public. IBE and ILAE work along with the World Health Organization (WHO) for a "Global Campaign against Epilepsy".

Epileptology took strong roots in Europe and North America after World War II and spread rapidly to other countries. In 1912, a second important drug, phenobarbitone, was introduced, which considerably improved the prospects of antiepileptic therapy. Around the late 1960s, there were three more effective antiepileptic drugs—(1) phenytoin, (2) carbamazepine, and (3) sodium valproate. With these four drugs, about 70% of the PWE can be made seizure free. With the availability of more drugs, the quality of life can be improved with reduction of side effects and better seizure control. Medical technology made rapid advances with long-term videos—EEG, CT, MRI, and positron emission tomography (PET), which help in better diagnosis. Along with drug treatment, neurosurgery is helping PWE for further improvement of life. From an "incurable" condition of earlier centuries, epilepsy today is an eminently treatable neurological disorder, which, however, still carries a totally unjustifiable social prejudice.

During the recent history on epilepsy, much work is being done worldwide through the initiative of the two premier organizations, ILAE and IBE both in view of medical research and social aspects. The European Association of Epilepsy Centers (EAECs) started functioning in 1988 in Zurich and spread to other parts of Europe under the initiative of people like Christoph Pachlatko (1956-2015), Harry Meinardi (1932-2013), and others.

The purpose of this association is to emphasize the unique structure and function of these centers differentiating them from the usual neurological and neuropediatric hospitals/departments in way of offering comprehensive care to the PWE.[6]

The European Forum on Epilepsy Research (ERF 2013), which started in Dublin, under the auspicious of ILAE and IBE, has identified the following projects on epilepsy research: (1) epilepsy in the developing brain, (2) novel targets for innovative diagnostics and treatment of epilepsy, (3) what is required for prevention and cure of epilepsy? and (4) epilepsy and comorbidities with focus on aging and mental health, with the motive to: (i) strengthen epilepsy research, (ii) reduce treatment gap, and (iii) reduce the burden and stigma associated with epilepsy.[7]

INDIAN SCENARIO

In the late 1960s, some senior Indian neurologists planned to start the Indian Epilepsy Association (IEA) independent of the Neurological Society of India (NSI) in order to accommodate nonmedical professionals for taking care of PWE. There was already an Epilepsy Section within the NSI, with Dr D Desai as secretary for the year 1968-1969. He along with Dr Eddie P Bharucha, Dr KS Mani, Dr Noshir H Wadia, and others, formed the IEA, independent of the NSI, which was registered on 21th March, 1970 in Bombay (now Mumbai).

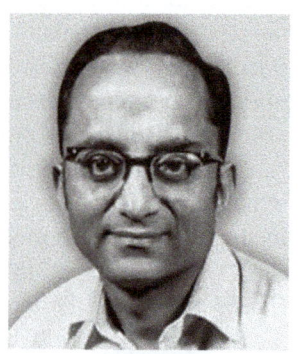

KS Mani

The IEA was affiliated to IBE in December 1974. Since then IEA chapters have grown all over India. The Bangalore chapter increased its membership rapidly with regular monthly meetings. Thanks to the dynamic leadership of KS Mani (1928-2001), whose inspiration leads the Bangalore chapter even today.

REFERENCES

1. Gabrielli F, Cocchi M, Levi D, et al. Historical-anthropological insights on epilepsy from Hippocrates to positivism. N Med. 2013;1:31-4.
2. Rai PV. Step by Step Treatment of Epilepsy. New Delhi: Jaypee Brothers Medical Publishers (P) Ltd; 2007.
3. Magiorkinis E, Diamantis A, Sidiropoulou K, et al. Highlights in the history of epilepsy: the last 200 years. Epilepsy Res Treat. 2014;2014:582039.
4. Jasper H, Penfield W. Epilepsy and the Functional Anatomy of the Human Brain, 2nd edition. United States: Little, Brown and Company; 1954.
5. Vishwanath RP, Christian S. Special Epilepsy Centers in Western Countries and Epilepsy Services in Developing Countries. Zurich: University of Zurich Publication; 1990.
6. Steinhoff BJ, Chatrou M, Hjalgrim H. Introduction: The European Association of Epilepsy Centers (EAEC). Epilepsy Behavior. 2017;76:S3.
7. Baulac M, de Boer H, Elger C, et al. Epilepsy priorities in Europe: A report of the ILAE-IBE Epilepsy Advocacy Europe Task Force. Epilepsia. 2015;56:1687-95.

2
Febrile Seizures

Subhas GT, Priyamvada Tatachar

INTRODUCTION

Febrile seizure is a seizure disorder exclusively occurring in childhood.

Febrile seizures are the most common type of seizures affecting 2-14% of children.

Although research supports most febrile seizures as being relatively benign, it is now accepted that a subgroup of children will experience consequences.

DEFINITION OF FEBRILE SEIZURES

A febrile seizure is defined as a seizure which is associated with fever and occurring in infants and children in the age group of 3 months to 5 years. There should not be any evidence of acute intracranial infection, defined cause, metabolic disturbance, or previous afebrile seizure. But the age group of onset may be advanced to 1 month of age (1 month to 5 years).[1]

The definition must be interpreted with caution as at times, especially in infants, seizures may occur even before the fever becomes obvious.

EPIDEMIOLOGY: BURDEN OF PROBLEMS

Although febrile seizure is seen in all ethnic groups, it is more frequently seen in the Asian population (5-10% of Indian children and 6-9% of Japanese children), with an incidence as high as 14% in Guam. The male-to-female ratio is approximately 1.6-1.8. Febrile seizures are more frequent among lower socioeconomic status and show a seasonal predilection to winter months.

ETIOLOGY: PREDISPOSING FACTORS—AGE

Febrile seizures are an age-dependent phenomenon, likely related to a vulnerability of the developing nervous system to the effects of fever in combination with an underlying genetic susceptibility. During the process of maturation there is an enhanced neuronal excitability that predisposes the child to febrile seizures.

FEVER—INFECTIONS

Seizures are usually precipitated when body temperature rises above 38°C rectally and usually occurs during the first 24 hours of febrile illness. But in some cases seizures occur before onset of fever. Extracranial infections like upper respiratory infection (URI), otitis media, gastroenteritis, pneumonia, urinary tract infection, viral infections commonly predispose infants and children to fever with higher temperatures and thereby to febrile seizures.

It is hypothesized that the presence of brain hyperexcitability with reduced seizure threshold and genetic predisposition is a cause for febrile seizure in infants and children.

IMMUNIZATION

Occasionally, febrile seizures may occur after administration of certain vaccines. The highest risk of febrile seizure is within 24 hours of receiving diphtheria, tetanus, and pertussis and 1-2 weeks of receiving mumps, measles, and rubella vaccines. The febrile seizures are the result of the fever, which follows vaccinations and not the vaccination itself. Newer acellular diphtheria/tetanus/pertussis is less reactogenic and there is a marked reduction in febrile seizures after vaccination. Genetic predisposition is also considered as the risk factor for genesis of febrile seizure in these children.

GENETICS

Genetic factors in association with environmental factors play an important role in occurrence of febrile seizures in many families. Polygenic inheritance with autosomal dominant presentation is seen in some families.

Mutations have been identified in sodium channel and in gamma-aminobutyric acid (GABA) receptor genes.

The probability of febrile seizures for a child is about 20% with an affected sibling with febrile seizure and it is more than 30% with affected parents and a sibling. The concordance rate is about 35-69% in monozygotic twins and 14-20% in dizygotic twins.

Generalized epilepsy with febrile seizures plus (GEFS+) syndrome, a familial epilepsy syndrome with variety of causative mutation, and Dravet syndrome [severe myoclonic epilepsy of infancy (SMEI)] though rare have a well-known preponderance for seizures with fever in early childhood and need to be considered in the differential diagnosis.

OTHER ASSOCIATED FACTORS

Premature birth, prenatal exposure to nicotine, and nutritional deficiencies especially iron, zinc, vitamin B12, folic acid, selenium, calcium, and manganese have been linked to development of febrile seizure.

Intrauterine growth retardation, neonatal intensive care unit stay >28 days, neurodevelopmental delay, and daycare attendance (due to predisposition to cross-infection) are considered as precipitating causes for febrile seizures.

CLINICAL FEATURES

Seizures occur early in the course of fever (<24 hours) and usually it is the first indicator of an underlying febrile illness. A febrile seizure occurs in significant proportion of occasions when the temperature is >38°C. Developing febrile seizures is dependent on the child's underlying seizure threshold and also genetic propensity.

CLASSIFICATIONS

Depending on the duration, repetition in the same febrile illness, and type (focal/generalized), febrile seizures are customarily classified as simple, complex, and febrile status epilepticus (FSE).

Simple febrile seizures are of short duration (10–15 minutes) mostly, but are not always generalized convulsions and do not repeat during the same febrile illness (24–48 hours). There is usually a brief postictal period and the child returns to normal without sequelae after the seizure. Simple febrile seizures constitute about 80% of febrile seizures. Children with simple febrile seizures have normal development.

Complex febrile seizures are febrile seizures with prolonged duration (most of the time) with focal features at the onset, recurring within 24 hours or within the same febrile illness (24–48 hours).

Transient hemiparesis following a febrile illness (Todd's paresis) may occur but is relatively rare. Children with complex febrile seizure are often younger (usually less than 1 year of age) and more likely to have abnormal development.[2]

There are a few criterias to differentiate simple and complex febrile seizures (Table 1).

Table 1: Differences between simple and complex febrile seizures.	
Simple febrile seizures	Complex febrile seizures
• Constitutes 80–85%	• Constitutes 15–20%
• Generalized tonic-clonic motor activity	• Focal seizures manifestation
• Seizure activity lasts <15 minutes with rapid return of consciousness	• Recurs more than once within 24 hours
• No postictal neurological abnormalities	• Postictal neurological abnormalities may be present
• Child having normal neurological and developmental status.	• Likely to have abnormal neurological status.

Febrile status epilepticus (FSE) is a continuous seizure or an intermittent seizure without neurological recovery lasting for 30 minutes or more, majority generalized tonic-clonic. Most seizures terminate spontaneously and the end is evidenced by a deep breath and closed eyes. Children with persistently open and deviated eyes might still be seizing despite cessation of convulsive activity. If the seizures fail to stop within 5 minutes, it is considered as prolonged seizure and if it continues in spite of acute therapy, it is also considered as FSE. FSE is rare but form significant proportion of the status epilepticus in children.

DIAGNOSTIC EVALUATION

A detailed history about the description of the seizures from the eyewitness and search for the cause of fever constitute the mainstay in the clinical evaluation of children with febrile seizures.

Clinical history includes questioning about:
- Seizure characteristics
- Duration of seizure
- Focality
- Personal or family history of seizure
- Immunization status and developmental status of the child.

A formal, general, and detailed neurological examination is done to identify the cause of fever and to detect the neurological abnormalities.

Neurological examination includes assessment of consciousness, muscle tone and power, deep tendon reflex, signs of meningeal irritation like neck stiffness, Kernig's signs, Brudzinski signs to rule out central nervous system (CNS) infection (meningitis, encephalitis), and check for impending sign of raised intracranial pressure like examination of fontanel (tense) and optic fundus (papilledema). Frequently meningitis initially presents with fever and seizure; however, in infants, these signs may not be present. Signs of head injury and markers of epilepsy (neurocutaneous markers) must be looked for. It is mandatory to evaluate neurological status serially.

DIFFERENTIAL DIAGNOSIS

This includes chills (shivering), febrile delirium, breath-holding spells, CNS infections (meningitis, encephalitis), febrile myoclonus, GEFS+ syndrome, Dravet syndrome (SMEI), and febrile infection-related epilepsy syndrome (FIRES).

Generalized epilepsy with febrile seizures plus is a familial epilepsy syndrome (SCNAIA, SCN2A, SCN1B, and GARBG2). It is an autosomal disorder with at least six phenotypes delineated by their causative genes. Initially seizures appear with fever but subsequently frequent febrile and afebrile seizures develop, which could be myoclonic, atonic, absence, or generalized tonic-clonic seizure (GTCS). Seizures with fever in GEFS+ continue beyond the age of 6 years.

Dravet syndrome is an autosomal dominant disorder due to de novo mutation. To start with, this epileptic syndrome of the infancy presents with prolonged febrile seizures, which may be unilateral. Subsequently, multiple prolonged afebrile seizures appear, which may be GTCS, myoclonic, partial, and are associated with psychomotor retardation. It is rare and described as SMEI.

A FIRES is a febrile infection-related epilepsy syndrome. A clinical entity present with status epilepticus following an infective event may be mistaken for FSE.

It is difficult to distinguish the first episode of the febrile seizure from a seizure resulting from epilepsy, GEFS+, SMEI, and FIRES in a child with fever. The diagnosis can only be made with evaluation of clinical symptomatology and laboratory investigations.

Investigative workup depends directly on the provisional diagnosis of febrile seizures. Basic workup is necessary to find out the causes of fever during the first simple febrile seizure, other investigations like metabolic workup, urine analysis (in case fever is obscure) are done. Depending upon the results of the clinical examination, lumbar puncture (LP) is mandatory in infants with first febrile seizure, when CNS infection is suspected or in those who are on prior antibiotic therapy and in FSE. LP should be considered in complex febrile seizures if neuroinfection is suspected. LP is not required in majority of the children with first simple febrile seizures.[3]

Electroencephalogram (EEG) is not useful in simple febrile seizures. It is rarely considered in complex febrile seizures when epilepsy is suspected.

Neuroimaging studies are not required in simple febrile seizures. Magnetic resonance imaging (MRI) (less preferably CT scan) should be considered in patients with signs of increase in intracranial pressure, with focal neurological abnormalities, suspected structural defects in the brain, abnormally large head, and in severe head injuries.

Genetic testing is not indicated in preliminary evaluation of febrile seizures. It should, however, be considered in patients where a genetic syndrome like Dravet syndrome is being considered on the basis of multiple prolonged febrile seizures.

TREATMENT OF FEBRILE SEIZURES IN ITS ACUTE PHASE

The majority of the febrile seizures end spontaneously by the time the child is first evaluated and the child usually returns quickly to normal baselines. In such cases, active treatment with benzodiazepines is not necessary. Fever should be treated symptomatically and causes of fever should be investigated.

There is no need for hospitalization. As with afebrile seizure, treatment should be started if the duration of seizures last for more than 5 minutes. Majority of the prolonged seizures are terminated by intravenous administration of lorazepam 0.1 mg/kg body weight at the rate of 2 mg/min or diazepam 0.2 mg/kg body weight at the rate of 1 mg/min to a maximum dose of 5 mg.

Close watch on breathing, arterial pulse and blood pressure should be monitored. If the seizure fails to stop, drugs may be repeated twice at 5 minutes interval.

If the intravenous route is inaccessible or unavailable in acute therapy, rectal administration of the diazepam (rectal preparation) in a single dose of 0.5 mg/kg body weight with option to repeat after 10 minutes or intranasal midazolam 0.2 mg/kg body weight (two puffs to each nostril) or 0.5 mg/kg body weight of midazolam is buccally recommended, and also in situations when the seizures are prolonged and no immediate medical care is available. These rescue medicines can be administered by parents at home and is safe and effective.

If immediate treatment of acute phase fails, the patient should be hospitalized and antiepileptic drugs (AEDs) should be administered. The line of management is the same as for afebrile status epilepticus and intravenous phenytoin/fosphenytoin, phenobarbitone, valproate, levetiracetam, and lacosamide are the preferred AEDs.

Hospital admission is considered when febrile seizures are prolonged and not terminated with acute therapy, when the seizures are focal, if there is delayed recovery to normal baseline status or when residual neurological defects are detected, and in all FSE. Hospitalization is also required to those suspected to have serious infections or other comorbidities.

RECURRENCE RISK

After the first febrile seizure, about one-third of the children in their early childhood will experience one or more recurrences but is relatively rare after 3 years of age.

The predictors for recurrences are:
- Age of onset in infancy or early childhood (<12–18 months)
- Low-grade fever during first febrile seizure
- Brief interval between seizure presentation and fever onset
- First febrile seizure presenting with features of complex febrile seizures
- Family history of febrile seizure (parent/siblings).

If none of the above predictive factors represent, the risk of recurrence of fever seizure is <15%.

In the presence of all the risk factors, the chances of recurrence febrile seizure may reach 80%. In spite of recurrence, simple febrile seizures are benign and will not have any effect on the growth and development in the affected children.[4]

PROPHYLAXIS

There are two types of prophylactic treatments:
1. Intermittent therapy
2. Continuous therapy.

Indications for Intermittent Therapy

Use of AEDs as prophylactic treatment is not justifiable when the natural history of febrile seizure is considered vis-à-vis when compared with risk following the use of AEDs.

But in a country like India where medical facilities in remote areas are not adequate or inaccessible, prophylactic treatment may have a role to play in children with prolonged febrile seizure or with a past history of complex febrile seizures.

In such situations, oral benzodiazepine (normally diazepam) is administered orally during febrile episode for 48 hours (0.33 mg/kg body weight, 8th hourly) and also may be given rectally (0.5 mg/kg body weight, 8th hourly). Other drugs commonly advised are oral preparation of clobazam during the first 48 hours of febrile episode (1 mg/kg body weight in two doses).

Indications for Continuous Therapy

Application of continuous AED treatment is not justifiable. Recurrences of febrile seizures are reduced with continuous therapy but are generally not considered worth the potential adverse effects of treatment.

The incidence of morbidity and mortality including FSE is rare without AED and has no impact on risk of latter epilepsy.

However, continuous AED therapy is rarely considered in patients with failed intermittent therapy or compulsion from anxious parents even after adequate counseling. If continuous AED is to be used, oral phenobarbitone is advocated (4 mg/kg body weight per day in two divided doses) and valproic acid is used very rarely. However, the risk and adverse effect of AEDs in personality development and behavioral disturbance with phenobarbitone and hepatotoxicity (hyperammonemia) of valproate outweigh the benefits. Unless barring compelling reasons, generally there is no role for prophylactic intermittent or continuous AED treatment in the management of febrile seizures.

Antipyretic drugs have no role in reducing the risk of febrile seizures or its recurrence. However, it may minimize the discomfort of the child during febrile episode. Oral paracetamol is the preferred antipyretic drug (20 mg/kg body weight in three doses) or ibuprofen (5 mg/kg body weight per dose) till the fever subsides (aspirin and nimesulide should be avoided). Tepid sponging to reduce the fever gives more discomfort to the child and is not recommended. An oral benzodiazepine and an oral antipyretic should be started at the onset of fever and have to be administered in every febrile episode till the child is 5 years of age.

PROGNOSIS

Neurologic sequel including new neurological defects, intellectual impairment, and behavioral abnormalities are rare following febrile seizures.

The risk of epilepsy in simple febrile seizure (about 2.5%) is marginally higher than in normal children.

The chances of development of epilepsy in febrile seizure under special circumstances like complex febrile seizure, FSE, with prior abnormal neurologic status or developmental impairment, family history of complex febrile seizure, or afebrile epilepsy are definitely more (>4%).

Febrile seizures do not appear to cause temporal lobe epilepsy. The association may represent an inherent susceptibility in some children who are predisposed to prolonged febrile seizures and epilepsy simultaneously.

Febrile status epilepticus is a rare event in febrile seizure, but forms a significant proportion of overall status epilepticus in children. FSE may present as first febrile seizure episodes or is more frequent in complex febrile seizures. Management of febrile status epilepsy with AEDs is in the same line as in the management of afebrile status epilepticus in children. Response to therapy is favorable. Subsequent development of epilepsy and mortality is rare.

To consider the abnormalities noticed in EEG and acute hippocampal injuries seen in MR imaging, postictally in FSE as the biomarker for future epilepsy is still to be confirmed.

PARENTAL COUNSELING

It is necessary to provide all the information about the natural history of febrile seizures to the parents soon after the first episode. Benign nature of the illness should be explained and parents should be properly counseled.

The importance of taking preventive measures to protect the child from contracting frequent infections should be highlighted.

At times, prolonged febrile seizures or multiple complex seizures may occur in short intervals and immediate medical aid may not be available. To face such situations, parents should be taught about administration of rescue medicines at home properly. They should be told to store thermometer, AEDs like diazepam (preferably rectal preparations), midazolam (nasal or buccal preparations), and antipyretic drugs (paracetamol oral) at home or while traveling.

They should also be sensitized about cardiopulmonary resuscitative procedures as first aid treatment and holding the child in semi-prone position to avoid aspiration during seizure episode.

The routine information about Do's and Don'ts during the seizure episode should be made available. Parents' doubts regarding subsequent neurological sequelae including appearance of new neurological deficits, intellectual impairment, and behavioral disorders following febrile seizures should be cleared.[5]

SUMMARY

Febrile seizures exclusively occur in infants and early childhood and are the most common seizure disorder in that age group.

Febrile seizures are genetically predetermined, age-dependent response to fever and are self-limited, prognosis is excellent, and risk of recurrence occurs in small proportion.

Risk of brain damage is extremely rare and simple febrile seizures do not adversely affect neurological status or mortality.

Severe recurrent attacks occur in less than 10% of febrile seizures and fewer than 5% develop epilepsy. Risk factors are identified to predict the recurrence after first febrile seizure and subsequent epilepsy. Application of diagnostic procedures depends upon the clinical assessment.

Treatment is initiated on selective basis. If a febrile seizure lasts for more than 5 minutes, it must be treated as a medical emergency.

Prophylactic therapy reduces recurrence and allays parental anxiety but does not prevent epilepsy. Parental counseling forms an important part of management of febrile seizures.

REFERENCES

1. Syndi Seinfeld D, Pellock JM. Recent research on febrile seizures: a review. J Neurol Neurophysiol. 2013;4:19519.
2. Leung AK. Febrile seizures. In: Leung AK (Ed). Common Problems in Ambulatory Pediatrics: Specific Clinical Problems. New York: Nova Science Publishers Inc.; 2011. pp. 199-206.
3. Subcommittee on Febrile Seizures, American Academy of Pediatrics. Neurodiagnostic evaluation of the child with a simple febrile seizure. Pediatrics. 2011;127(2):389-94.
4. Nelson KB, Ellenberg JH. Predictors of epilepsy in children who have experienced febrile seizure. N Engl J Med. 1976;295(19):1029-33.
5. Khair AM, Elmagrabi D. Febrile seizures and febrile seizure syndromes: an updated overview of old and current knowledge. Neurol Res Int. 2015; 2015:849341.

3
Epilepsy and Epilepsy Syndromes in Children

Raghavendra K

INTRODUCTION

Childhood epilepsies have heterogeneous but unique characteristics with respective semiology, pharmacological responsiveness, and prognosis, which differentiate them from adult-onset epilepsies.[1,2] This warrants a multiaxial diagnostic approach to childhood epilepsies. Also, many causes of symptomatic epilepsies such as malformations of cortical development as well as epileptic encephalopathy (EE) syndrome are relatively specific to the pediatric population. The immature brain is susceptible to many unfavorable conditions such as hypoxia, prolonged epileptiform activity (e.g. status epilepticus), or brain inflammation, which is highly age-dependent as per the theory of critical developmental periods. Moreover, the phenotypic characteristics of epilepsy, such as seizure type and sensitivity to treatments, can change with maturation.[3,4]

EPIDEMIOLOGY

Epilepsy is one of the most common pediatric neurologic disorders with up to 0.5–1.0%, of children less than 16 years, being affected with it. The median incidence of epilepsy in childhood (0–14 years) is higher than the adult population (82/100,000/year vs. 34.7/100,000/year).[5] The incidence of new-onset epilepsy in children in the general population is about five cases per 10,000 per year with 23–33% of them having the likelihood of becoming pharmacoresistant. The incidence of different types of seizures is also seen to vary as compared to adult population.[3,4,6]

Idiopathic (genetic) epilepsy, both focal and generalized seizures, constitutes approximately 30% of new-onset epilepsies in children. Symptomatic (structural-metabolic) epilepsies, which are identified by the presence of a neurological deficit or structural abnormalities on neuroimaging, constitute 20% of all new-onset pediatric epilepsy cases. Only 11–35% of pediatric population with positive MRI scans have the likelihood of becoming seizure free with medication. The major proportion of new-onset seizures in children is cryptogenic (unknown) epilepsies. These are epilepsies in which the cause cannot be detected with the currently available methods of evaluation.[7] However, this proportion is progressively declining with advances in investigative modalities that have helped in detection of complex genetic or microstructural abnormalities.[8,9]

APPROACH TO CHILD WITH SEIZURE

It is recommend to approach the child suspected with epilepsy with the following progressive axis:[3]
- Is it truly "epilepsy"?
- Can the seizure be classified into a particular type?
- Can the epilepsy be classified into a particular syndrome?
- Is there any underlying cause for the epilepsy?
- What are the associated comorbidities?

Is It Truly "Epilepsy"?

While making a diagnosis of epilepsy in children, a number of paroxysmal conditions, which can resemble an epileptic seizure, are to be borne in mind. Failure to recognize them lead to a misdiagnosis, which has been shown to be as high as 39%. The accurate description of the episode or episodes by the patient and witnesses can help in differentiation of an epileptic or nonepileptic event.[1]

The most common mimics of childhood epilepsy and age-related differential diagnosis are depicted in Tables 1 and 2.

Table 1: Common nonepileptic paroxysmal events by age.[1]	
Newborn	• Jitteriness • Benign sleep myoclonus • Hyperekplexia
Infancy and early childhood	• Breath-holding spells • Shuddering attacks • Stereotypes • Benign paroxysmal torticollis • Benign paroxysmal tonic upward gaze • Benign paroxysmal vertigo • Sleep disorders • Masturbation (gratification behaviors) • Spasmus nutans • Sandifer syndrome • Tics
Adolescent	• Syncope • Sleep disorders • Psychogenic crises • Tics • Migraine

Source: Modified from Tatlı B, Güler S. Çocukluk Çağında Non Epileptik Paroksismal Olaylar. Turk Pediatr Ars. 2017;52(2):59-65.

Table 2: Nonepileptic paroxysmal events (NEPEs) and the epileptic conditions that they imitate.[1]	
NEPE	Imitating epileptic conditions
Syncope	Generalized tonic-clonic seizures, focal seizures, absence seizures, drop attacks, and myoclonic seizures
Breath-holding spell	Tonic spasms
Sandifer syndrome	Tonic spasms, infantile spasm
Sleep disorders	Frontal lobe seizures, rolandic seizure
Benign sleep myoclonus	Myoclonic seizure, focal seizures
Pseudocrisis	Status epilepticus, nonconvulsive status, tonic-clonic seizures, absence seizures, and focal seizures
Migraine	Occipital lobe seizures, temporal lobe seizures

Source: Modified from Tatlı B, Güler S. Çocukluk Çağında Non Epileptik Paroksismal Olaylar. Turk Pediatr Ars. 2017;52(2):59-65.

What are the Seizure Types?

Whenever a child presents with seizure, every attempt should be made to get a clear description of the event(s) so as to classify them into the appropriate seizure type. The seizure description must be evaluated for a generalized or a focal onset. A focal onset can be further lateralized to a hemisphere or localized to a lobe. The details of description of the seizure types as per the International League Against Epilepsy (ILAE) are given in Box 1.

Can the Epilepsy be Classified into a Particular Syndrome?

Epilepsy syndrome as per the ILAE is defined as a distinctive disorder identifiable on the basis of a typical age of onset, specific electroencephalogram (EEG) characteristics, seizure types, and other features. Multiple epilepsy syndromes are recognized by the ILAE and this syndrome classification is very important in children as it enables the clinician to consider relevant investigations and direct treatment choice in addition to avoiding medications, which are known to exacerbate the seizures. It also allows prognostication regarding the likely future course of the epilepsy to the child and family. The seizure syndrome classification takes seizure types, age of onset, distinctive comorbidities including intellectual and psychiatric dysfunction along with specific EEG, and imaging findings. There are multiple clinicoelectrophysiological syndromes that have been recommended, of which 31 epilepsy syndromes have been described by the ILAE.[8]

The clinicoelectrographic description with treatment and prognosis of the commonly encountered syndromes are provided in Tables 3A and B.

Box 1: Classification of seizure types.[3]
- *Generalized seizures (arising within and rapidly engaging bilaterally distributed networks):*
  - Tonic-clonic
  - Clonic
  - Absence including typical, atypical and absence with special features such as myoclonic absence, eyelid myoclonia
  - Tonic
  - Atonic
  - Myoclonic
  - Unknown epileptic spasms
- *Focal seizures (originating within networks limited to one hemisphere):* It can be classified by features, and/or laterality and/or lobar localization.
  - *Characterized by features (clinical)*: One or more types of features may be present during any single focal seizure including aura, motor manifestation, autonomic manifestation, and presence or absence of awareness/responsiveness.
  - *By hemispheric localization (clinical or electrophysiological)*: Right or left. Based on lateralizing features such as head turning, eye deviation, and unilateral clonic movements, all lateralize to the contralateral hemisphere.
  - *By lobar localization (clinical or electrophysiological)*: Frontal/temporal/occipital/parietal/insular lobe.
    For example, frontal lobe seizures are usually brief. Motor features are prominent. There may be vocalization, bizarre behavior, head and eye deviation, and urinary incontinence.
- *Epileptic spasms*: With specific semiology in the form of seizure characterized by sudden flexion, extension, or mixed flexion-extension of proximal and truncal muscles, lasting 1-2 seconds and can be bilaterally symmetric, asymmetric, or unilateral.

ETIOLOGY

The previous ILAE etiological categorization of seizures into "idiopathic", "symptomatic", and "cryptogenic" has been replaced by better precise terms such as "genetic", "structural", and "metabolic" to which "immune" and "infectious" etiologies have been added recently. This classification holds true for the pediatric population as well.[3,8]

- *Structural etiology*: Epilepsies with structural abnormality are visible on structural neuroimaging with supportive electroclinical findings as likely cause of seizures. This includes acquired causes such as stroke, trauma, and infection as well as genetic causes along with malformations of cortical development. The mesial temporal lobe seizures with Rasmussen syndrome, hippocampal sclerosis, hypothalamic hamartoma, and hemiconvulsion-hemiplegia epilepsy and other commonly associated structural lesions.[1,4,8,10]
- *Genetic etiology*: Here the epilepsy is either a direct result or a presumed genetic mutation in which seizures are the core symptom of the disorder.

Table 3A: Epilepsy syndromes occurring during early childhood.

Epilepsy syndromes	Age at onset	Etiology	Seizure types	EEG findings	Treatment	Outcome
Benign familial neonatal seizures	First week of life (2nd or 3rd day) Boys = Girls	Autosomal dominant channelopathy—KCNQ2 and KCNQ3	Brief, frequent (20–30/day), tonic motor activity and posturing with apnea, vocalizations, ocular symptoms, motor automatisms, chewing, focal or generalized clonic movements, and clonic components of the later phase are usually asymmetrical and unilateral	• *Interictal EEG:* Normal or discontinuous with or without focal or multifocal abnormalities or theta pointu alternant pattern • *Ictal EEG:* Synchronous and bilateral flattening of 5–19 seconds coinciding with apnea and tonic motor activity	• Remit spontaneously without medication	Prognosis is good
Benign neonatal seizures (nonfamilial)	Between days 1 and 7 of life 90%, between 4 days and 6 days—"5th day fits" Common in boys	Environmental	Clonic status epilepticus in the form of successive unilateral clonic convulsions affecting predominantly the face and limbs with frequent change sides, less often bilateral, concomitant apnea. Tonic seizures are incompatible with this syndrome	• *Interictal EEG* shows a "theta pointu alternant pattern" • *Ictal EEG:* Rhythmic spikes or slow waves in the rolandic regions, although they can also localize anywhere.	• Remit spontaneously without medication • Prolonged seizures IV benzodiazepines and phenytoin.	Commonly excellent
Benign familial infantile seizures	3–8 months Strong family history	Genetically heterogeneous disease—PRRT2, SCN2A, KCNQ2, and KCNQ3	Focal clusters, brief episodes of motor arrest, unresponsiveness, head and/or eye deviation to one side, staring, fluttering of eyelids, grunting, and cyanosis	• *Interictal EEG:* Normal, ictal EEG—partial seizures originate from the parietal-occipital region • Variation of the side of hemisphere between episodes.	Antiepileptic treatment with carbamazepine, valproate, and phenobarbital	Prognosis is good

(EEG: electroencephalogram; IV: intravenous)

Table 3B: Benign or self-limiting focal epilepsy syndromes of later childhood and adolescence.

Epilepsy syndromes	Age at onset	Etiology	Seizure types	EEG findings	Treatment	Outcome
Benign childhood epilepsy with centrotemporal spikes (BCECTS)	7 years and 10 years (peak 8 years or 9 years)	• Genetically determined • AD inheritance with age-dependent penetrance.	Hemifacial and oropharyngolaryngeal sensorimotor seizures—numbness, paraesthesias, strange sounds (gargling, grunting and guttural sounds, and combinations), speech arrest, and hypersalivation. Secondary generalization in 50%	• *Interictal EEG:* High amplitude, sharp and slow-wave complexes localized—C3–C4 (central) or C5–C6 (midway between central and temporal) • *Ictal:* Rare ipsilateral rolandic regions and consists of slow waves mixed with fast rhythms and spikes.	Carbamazepine, levetiracetam	Invariably excellent
Panayiotopoulos syndrome	3–6 years of age (peak 4 years or 5 years)	Probably genetically determined	Constellation of autonomic, mainly emetic, symptoms, behavioral changes, unilateral deviation of the eyes. Consciousness and speech are preserved at seizure onset. Autonomic features (81%)—emetic (72%), pallor, flushing, or cyanosis; mydriasis, miosis; hypersalivation, cardiorespiratory, and thermoregulatory alterations; coughing; urinary and/or fecal incontinence; and modifications of intestinal motility. Headaches (cephalic auras) may occur at onset	• *Interictal EEG:* Multifocal, high amplitude, sharp slow-wave complexes, spikes. – Can be widely distributed, often shifting from one region to another – Sleep accentuation is present. • *Ictal EEG:* Slow activity with spikes.	Education key AED rarely needed prophylactic treatment only if prolonged autonomic status epilepticus	Excellent

Contd...

Contd...

Epilepsy syndromes	Age at onset	Etiology	Seizure types	EEG findings	Treatment	Outcome
Idiopathic childhood occipital epilepsy of Gastaut	3 years and 15 years (peak around 8 years)	Unclear	• Purely occipital manifestation with elementary visual hallucinations, blindness or both, deviation of the eyes, forced eyelid closure, and eyelid blinking • Complex visual hallucinations, visual illusions and other symptoms, postictal headache.	• *Interictal EEG:* Occipital paroxysms with fixation-off sensitivity • *Ictal EEG:* Preceded by regression of occipital paroxysms, followed by sudden appearance of occipital discharges consisting of spikes and fast rhythms.	Carbamazepine with slow reduction in the dose of medication of 2 years or 3 years	Remission 50–60%

(AED: antiepileptic drug; EEG: electroencephalogram)

Genetic basis to seizure may be based on family history, clinical research, and/or through identification implicated gene or genes or through detection of copy number variant in genes with major effect.
- *Infectious etiology*: Most common etiology worldwide including India. The most common cause being neurocysticercosis, followed by meningitis and acute meningoencephalitis.
- *Metabolic etiology*: Here the epilepsy may dominate the clinical picture and be a common feature in several inborn errors of metabolism (IEM). They share certain clinical features of presentation at early agency—morbid developmental delay/regression along with extraneurologic findings and seizures often being resistant to conventional antiepileptic drug (AED) therapy. Identifying specific metabolic causes of epilepsy becomes extremely important in view of the availability of specific therapies, which not only help in controlling the seizure but also in preventing potential intellectual impairment.[11,12]
- *Immune etiology*: Immune epilepsies with seizures as core symptom arise due to direct immune-mediated mechanisms and include autoimmune epilepsy and few of the epileptic encephalopathies. Seizures are common in limbic encephalitis or multifocal paraneoplastic disorders. N-methyl-D-aspartate (NMDA) receptor and leucine-rich glioma-inactivated 1 (LGI-1) encephalitis are highly associated with seizures. It is critical to diagnose this etiologic subgroup since specific category-targeted immunotherapies are available.[8]
- *Developmental and epileptic encephalopathies*: The term developmental encephalopathy is used when there is just developmental impairment without frequent epileptic activity associated with regression or further slowing of development. The term EE is used when there is no pre-existing developmental delay and the genetic mutation is not thought to cause slowing in its own right. EE is a term used when the epileptic activity itself contributes to severe cognitive and behavioral deficits, which is above and beyond that might be explained from the underlying pathology alone. Developmental and epileptic encephalopathies are used together when both factors play a role. These are the special types of epileptic syndromes, which are almost restricted to childhood and can have a devastating impact. The cognitive or behavioral impairment can be global or selective, and generally tends to worsen with time. EE usually has a well-defined age of seizure onset, characteristic seizure semiology, frequency, duration, underling etiological/inciting factors, as well as characteristic findings on EEG.[8]

SPECIAL CONDITIONS IN CHILDREN

- *Febrile seizures (FSs)*: As per the American Academy of Pediatrics (AAP), febrile seizures are currently defined as seizures occurring in febrile children between the ages of 6 months and 60 months who do not have an intracranial infection, metabolic disturbance, or history of afebrile seizures. The basic pathophysiology proposed is genetic predisposition, which results in neurodevelopmental vulnerability that has been hypothesized to be due to single or multiple factors including altered expression in sodium channel, hypothalamic dysregulation, and alteration in cortical or/and hippocampal excitability. The environmental triggers further modify these factors to cause seizures through neurotropicity and metabolic dysregulatory pathways.

Generally, cut-off point is when the body temperature rises above 38°C rectally. The peak incidence is between 18 months and 22 months of age. FSs are further classified into simple (generalized, single episode during one febrile episode) and complex (focal, multiple during the febrile illness, prolonged, lasting >15 minutes). Epidemiological studies show that 2% of infants with simple FS and 4–12% with complex FS develop epilepsy in later life. The frequency of developing epilepsy may ranging from 2 times to 18 times that of the general population resulting due to the different genetic basis of simple FS and complex FS. Presence of neurological abnormalities along with developmental delays is often associated with higher risk of FS. The best treatment policy is to educate the parents regarding the benign nature of the illness and also the risks and benefits associated with medication. Long-term management of FS includes two types of therapy—(1) intermittent medication at the time of fever and (2) daily (continuous) medications.[3]

- *Symptomatic focal epilepsy—focal epileptogenic lesions*: The spectrum of focal epileptogenic lesions and their clinical manifestations differ significantly among the pediatric age group as compared to adults. This includes unique causes like large hemispheric lesions, neurocutaneous syndromes, and developmental brain tumors. Symptomatic focal epilepsies consist of a wide range of lesions varying from congenital lesions such as malformations of cortical development (MCD) (like dysplasia/polymicrogyria) and developmental tumors [ganglioglioma, dysembryoplastic neuroepithelial tumors (DNETs)] to lesions such as encephalomalacia, which are acquired due to a variety of brain injuries. In addition, the likelihood of the mesial temporal sclerosis (MTS) having a dual pathology among children is also high. The importance of this group is that they are highly refractory and are also candidates for surgical evaluation. In infancy, the semiology of seizure may be more generalized with more diffuse and nonlocalizing EEG abnormalities.[3,8,10]

- *Malformations of cortical development*: With recent advances in imaging, molecular, genetic, and histopathological analysis, the MCD has emerged as a leading major category of disorders associated with pediatric epilepsy with majority of this category being medical intractability to therapy.

Malformations of cortical development are a diverse group of developmental disorders resulting as a result of defect or insult during various stage of normal cortical development including cellular proliferation and differentiation, neuronal migration, and cortical organization. Based on the stage of cortical development that is primarily disrupted, they are further classified. The subgroup of MCD that arises due to defects in the proliferative stage of cortical development is likely to be associated with medically intractable epilepsy with focal cortical dysplasia with balloon cells, tuberous sclerosis complex, hemimegalencephaly, and ganglioglioma as few examples.[8,10]

- *Hypothalamic hamartomas (HHs)*: These are rare benign developmental malformations occurring in the region of the tuber cinereum and third ventricle with close resemblance to a normal hypothalamus. They have the ability of intrinsic subcortical epileptogenesis and are frequently associated with drug-resistant intractable seizures, cognitive impairment, behavioral disturbances, and endocrinal abnormalities including central precocious puberty. The hallmark of HH being gelastic seizures, which occur in early age with development of additional seizure types later on. Symptomatic epilepsy in HH is an indication for surgical resection. Individualizing the treatment plan may be needed for each patient depending on the experience and comfort level of the treating physician with these techniques.[8,10]
- *Generalized epilepsy with febrile seizures plus (GEFS+)*: GEFS+, an idiopathic epilepsy syndrome, is a group of epilepsy syndromes that are inherited in an autosomal dominant fashion with incomplete penetrance. The classical hallmark presentation is febrile seizures in infancy or early childhood, which later develops into epilepsy with various seizure types, such as generalized tonic-clonic, absence, or myoclonic seizure. There will be a strong association of a history of a mixture of FSs and other seizure types among family members.

Even though many genes have been identified that are associated with GEFS+, the *SCN1A* gene mutation has the focus of attention. The clinical manifestation includes a spectrum of subtle FSs to catastrophic epilepsy syndrome such as Dravet syndrome depending on the gene as well as the type of genetic abnormalities.[8]

COMORBIDITY OF CHILDHOOD EPILEPSY

Pediatric epilepsy is said to be a developmental neuropsychiatric disorder with behavioral, cognitive, and linguistic comorbidities as manifestations of the disorder in addition to seizures.

Comorbid conditions may be more disabling and difficult to manage than the seizures themselves and, hence it is recommended that these comorbidities are looked for not only at initial evaluation but also during follow-up after treatment.[2,3,8,9]

In population-based studies, 70–76% of children with epilepsy are known to suffer from some type of disability or handicap, thus influencing future choices.

- *Neurological comorbidities*: Cognitive impairment, language impairment, migraine, and sleep problems are major comorbidities. The intellectual disability is the most common comorbidity occurring in up to 30–40% and is more common in the devastating epilepsy syndromes such as infantile spasms, Dravet syndrome, and Lennox-Gastaut syndrome.

Cognitive impairment is also observed in the so-called "benign epilepsy" like absence epilepsy. Children with symptomatic generalized epilepsy performed worse than idiopathic generalized epilepsy and focal epilepsy. Presence of abnormal EEGs lowered the IQ score as compared to normal EEG.

Language impairment is observed in up to 27.5% and can extend from basic to higher level linguistic deficits. Landau-Kleffner syndrome (LKS) and the epilepsy with continuous spike waves during slow-wave sleep (CSWS) are two of the specific epilepsy syndromes that are associated with language impairment as presentation.

Children with epilepsy have a wide spectrum of problems related to sleep including parasomnias, alteration of sleep architecture-like sleep fragmentation, daytime drowsiness, and bedtime difficulties.

- *Psychiatric comorbidities*: Autism-spectrum disorders, attention-deficit/hyperactivity disorder (ADHD), mood disorders, depressive and anxiety disorders, oppositional defiant and psychosis, and tic disorders to lesser extent are associated with epilepsy.

Families with children suffering with epilepsy are more likely to suffer from psychosocial and familial problems. In addition, they are also likely to share medical problems similar to adults such as bone loss, immunological disturbances, somatic growth abnormalities, and endocrine and metabolic abnormalities (hypothyroidism, growth hormone deficiency, polycystic ovary syndrome and sexual maturation-related issues, and dyslipidemia as well as secondary carnitine deficiency), many of which may be AED related.

MANAGEMENT

Management of childhood epilepsy requires a holistic approach, which includes understanding of the syndrome, comorbidity as well as of pharmacokinetics, including drug metabolic interaction in case of polytherapy. Regular monitoring for toxicity during follow-up is required. The family members are advised to seek medical attention at the earliest, if there are any potential side effects.[1,8]

In children, after the decision to start the medication is taken, one should plan the required sequence of drugs that are appropriate for the given syndrome. This is after assessment of benefit/risk ratio of the drug for that particular condition and also including the drug-specific cognitive impact. Early intervention to control seizures is necessary not only for abating serious neurodevelopmental consequences, but is also critical to reducing seizure-related morbidity and mortality.[4]

The issues of age-dependent effects of pharmacokinetics, tolerability, age-dependent efficacy, and worsening effect of drugs have to be borne in mind before initiation of AEDs in children, especially in infants. Also, the child should be managed by a multidisciplinary team so not only the child's epilepsy-related needs but also the associated comorbidities are addressed.[8]

Up to 60% achieve complete seizure freedom on a therapeutic dose of the appropriately chosen first AED. Evidence-based approach should be adopted for choice of AED in focal or generalized seizures or even in etiology-specific or syndrome-based treatment. For epilepsy with focal seizures, as per the SANAD trial, lamotrigine and carbamazepine have been more efficacious than gabapentin and topiramate with a smaller side effect profile in lamotrigine. For epilepsy with generalized seizures, sodium valproate is outperformed. Topiramate and lamotrigine are well-tolerated.[8]

In few conditions, etiology-specific therapy can be offered especially in many of the rare inherited metabolic diseases such as pyridoxine dependency and glucose transporter type 1 (GLUT1) deficiency syndrome.[11,12]

PEDIATRIC INTRACTABLE EPILEPSY SYNDROMES

Even with the discovery of newer AEDs, up to 40% of childhood epilepsy patients fail to achieve seizure freedom leading to a devastating effect on the child as well as the caregiver. Hence, it is imperative that refractory epilepsy is recognized early so as to minimize the consequences including mortality due to pharmacoresistant epilepsy (which is up to 4/1,000 person years). During the evaluation of pediatric epilepsy, predictors of development of refractory seizures such as presence of mental retardation, perinatal anoxia, neonatal convulsions, status epilepticus, and symptomatic etiology have to be enquired. Younger age of onset, higher initial seizure frequency, focal EEG, seizure onset under 1 year of age as well as multiple seizure types are early markers of intractability. All subjects with refractory seizures or children with conditions that predisposes refractory epilepsy (like MCD) should be referred to a specialist epilepsy center for further evaluation for possible search of surgical candidates. Long-term seizure freedom following epilepsy surgery can be achieved in up to 30–80% of pediatric population on detection of such surgically amendable lesions. For nonsurgical pathologies, nonresective palliative surgical options including interhemispheric disconnection, multiple subpial transections, and vagal nerve stimulation (VNS) can be explored. Interhemispheric disconnection is especially show to influence the falls (drop attacks) that are associated with many catastrophic seizure syndromes. VNS is another surgical option that is available when possibility of targeted lesional treatment is excluded. In recent studies, newer surgical modalities such as deep brain stimulation are showing promising evidence and may need to be explored further in pediatric population.[3,4,9]

When epilepsy surgery is not an option, alternatives such as ketogenic diet should be explored. Seizure reduction of >50% has been reported. Modern forms of ketogenic diet such as the modified Atkins diet almost as equally as efficacious as add-on AED therapy.[4]

CONCLUSION

Pediatric epilepsy syndromes are a conglomerate of disorders with a wide variety of causes and clinical presentations different from adult-onset epilepsies. In addition to the seizures, the quality of life is impaired by cognitive and psychiatric comorbidities. Hence, there should be a multiaxial approach for establishing diagnosis through structured approach for seizure control as well as for improvement in the quality of life. Epilepsy classification in children is distributed over a spectrum of disorders many of which are age-dependent. Even though seizure freedom is achieved in majority of children with appropriately chosen single AED, a significant proportionate of them are refractory epilepsy cases. These may be additionally helped with surgical options. With recent advances in genetic and imaging understanding of pediatric epilepsy, a subject-specific personalized approach of management may be the future.

REFERENCES

1. Tatlı B, Güler S. Çocukluk Çağında Non Epileptik Paroksismal Olaylar. Turk Pediatr Ars. 2017;52(2):59-65.
2. Kotsopoulos IA, Van Merode T, Kessels FG, et al. Systematic review and meta-analysis of incidence studies of epilepsy and unprovoked seizures. Epilepsia. 2002;43(11):1402-9.
3. Zuberi SM, Symonds JD. Atualização sobre o diagnóstico e tratamento de epilepsias da infância. J Pediatr. 2015;91(6):S67-77.
4. Berg AT. Identification of pharmacoresistant epilepsy. Neurol Clin. 2009;27(4):1003-13.
5. Sanchez RM, Jensen FE. Maturational aspects of epilepsy mechanisms and consequences for the immature brain. Epilepsia. 2001;42(5):577-85.
6. Gadgil P, Udani V. Pediatric epilepsy: the Indian experience. J Pediatr Neurosci. 2011;6(Suppl 1):S126-9.
7. Reif PS, Tsai MH, Helbig I, et al. Precision medicine in genetic epilepsies: break of dawn? Expert Rev Neurother. 2017;17(4):381-92.

8. Boller OI, Swaab DF. Pediatric Neurology. In: Aminoff MJ, Swaab DF (Eds). Handbook of Clinical Neurology. New York: Elsevier; 2018.
9. Shinnar S, Pellock JM. Update on the epidemiology and prognosis of pediatric epilepsy. J Child Neurol. 2002;17 Suppl 1:S4-17.
10. Barkovich AJ, Guerrini R, Kuzniecky RI, et al. A developmental and genetic classification for malformations of cortical development: update 2012. Brain. 2012;135(Pt 5):1348-69.
11. Rahman S, Footitt EJ, Varadkar S, et al. Inborn errors of metabolism causing epilepsy. Dev Med Child Neurol. 2013;55(1):23-36.
12. Thomas B, Al Dossary N, Widjaja E. MRI of childhood epilepsy due to inborn errors of metabolism. Am J Roentgenol. 2010;194(5):W367-74.

4

New-onset Epilepsy in Adults

Delon D'Souza, Thomas Mathew

INTRODUCTION

Epilepsy is defined as a disorder of the brain characterized by an enduring predisposition to generate epileptic seizures. It has been defined as two or more unprovoked seizures occurring more than 24 hours apart or one unprovoked seizure and a high risk (at least 60%) of recurrent unprovoked seizures over the next 10 years.[1] In this chapter, we will be focusing on adults (18–65 years) with epilepsy.

Before making a diagnosis of epilepsy, it is imperative that one should rule out other causes of impaired consciousness or involuntary movements. These include syncope, hypoglycemia, transient ischemic attacks, nonepileptic attacks, complicated migraine, movement disorders such as paroxysmal dyskinesia, or sleep disorders to name a few. In elderly adults, one important differential diagnosis is syncope, especially cardiogenic syncope. Patients can have temporary loss of consciousness due to cerebral hypoperfusion. The onset may be abrupt or gradual. Patient may describe a feeling of lightheadedness at onset. It may be accompanied by sweating or cold extremities and blurring of vision (presyncope). Symptoms are precipitated by upright position, exertion, or emotional stress. As the patient slumps to the ground, there may be a brief loss of consciousness. However, if the syncope is prolonged either due to upright posture or sustained arrhythmia, patient may develop myoclonic jerks or rarely tonic-clonic movements (convulsive syncope). Urinary incontinence or tongue bite may occur in syncope also. In these situations, patients may be mistakenly treated as epilepsy whereas fatal arrhythmias or heart blocks may be the real cause of recurrent loss of consciousness. Therefore, it is important to take a detailed firsthand account of events preceding the episode of loss of consciousness both from the patient and witness. If an episode is witnessed, record the pulse and blood pressure during the episode and get an urgent electrocardiogram (ECG) done. Holter monitoring or autonomic function tests may be required when there is a high index of suspicion for syncope. In younger patients, episodes of vasovagal syncope precipitated by emotional stress, fatigue, or anxiety may be similarly mistaken for epilepsy.

The diagnosis of seizure is largely made on clinical grounds supported by imaging and electroencephalogram (EEG) findings.

Provoking factors and secondary causes should be excluded before focusing on epilepsy. Patients with new-onset epilepsy may present with any seizure type. Most common seizure types seen are generalized tonic-clonic seizures (GTCS), focal seizures with or without impaired awareness, and focal to bilateral tonic-clonic seizures. Most provoked seizures present with GTCS. However, it is important to identify subtle clinical symptoms that precede the GTCS (aura), which give a clue to focal onset of the epilepsy.

Juvenile myoclonic epilepsy (JME) and mesial temporal lobe sclerosis (MTLS) are the two important epileptic syndromes that may occur during adulthood. Apart from these two epileptic syndromes, in most other epilepsies in adults, we may have to rule out a secondary cause. Careful evaluation of the provoking factors is a must to conclude that a seizure is truly unprovoked. Sleep deprivation, video games, essential oils such as eucalyptus, camphor, and drugs can be a provoking factor for seizure, which should be ruled out before labeling the seizure unprovoked or idiopathic. Hypoglycemia, hyperglycemia, hyponatremia, and hypocalcemia can also cause recurrent seizures and can be an important cause for new-onset epilepsy in adults (NOEA). Autoimmune encephalopathies secondary to various autoimmune antibodies such as anti-Leucine-rich Glioma-Inactivated 1 (anti-LGI1), anti-N-methyl-D-aspartate (anti-NMDA), and anti-gamma-aminobutyric acid (anti-GABA) receptor antibodies can cause NOEA. NOEA may be true new-onset epilepsy in adulthood (occurring after the age of 18 years) or continuing into adulthood after having onset in childhood or adolescence.

New-onset epilepsy in adults (includes both GTCS and focal seizure) can be broadly classified as primary and secondary, the causes for which are given in Table 1.

PRIMARY NEW-ONSET EPILEPSY IN ADULTS

Most genetic/idiopathic epilepsies have their onset in childhood and adolescence. Two important epileptic syndromes that may have onset in adulthood are: (1) JME and (2) MTLS.[2]

Juvenile Myoclonic Epilepsy

Juvenile myoclonic epilepsy is classically described with an onset in adolescence. However, it can manifest in adult life and is usually undiagnosed for a long time. Studies have shown a delay of 6.3–15 years in the diagnosis of JME in both developed and developing countries.[3] JME is characterized by GTCS with myoclonic jerks that occur in the early hours after awakening from sleep. Myoclonic jerks are brief shock-like

Table 1: Causes of primary and secondary NOEA.	
Primary NOEA	
Genetic/idiopathic	Juvenile myoclonic epilepsy and mesial temporal lobe sclerosis
Secondary NOEA	
Infections	Tuberculosis, cysticercal granuloma, herpes encephalitis, HIV, and neurosyphilis
Structural	Post-traumatic, poststroke, tumors, arteriovenous malformations, cavernous angiomas, malformations of cortical development such as focal cortical dysplasia
Metabolic	Hyperglycemia, hypoglycemia, hyponatremia, hypernatremia, and hypocalcemia
Inflammatory/autoimmune	ADEM, vasculitis, autoimmune encephalitis, SLE, and CNS vasculitis
Drugs	Tramadol, quinolones, ephedrine, phenylephrine, and linezolid
Essential oil-related seizure	Eucalyptus, camphor, and their combinations
Neurodegenerative/mitochondrial/storage disorders	SCA7, SCA10, MERRF, adult-onset neuronal ceroid-lipofuscinosis (NCL), and Alzheimer's dementia

(ADEM: acute disseminated encephalomyelitis; CNS: central nervous system; HIV: human immunodeficiency virus; MERRF: myoclonic epilepsy with ragged-red fibers; NOEA: new-onset epilepsy in adults; SLE: systemic lupus erythematosus)

contractions seen predominantly in the upper limb and trunk. One-third of the patients also have absence seizures. Absence seizures in JME are mild and often go unnoticed. The seizures, especially myoclonic jerks, occur due to sleep deprivation. MRI of brain is normal and EEG shows generalized spike, polyspike, and wave discharges. Photoparoxysmal response is seen in one-third of the patients. Only few patients have clinical photosensitive seizures. The EEG abnormalities are more pronounced if done after sleep deprivation and with adequate photic stimulation. There are documented cases of EEG showing focal discharges or asymmetry in the epileptiform discharges in JME. Hence, a strong clinical suspicion is required, especially when a patient is refractory to treatment with sodium channel blockers like phenytoin and carbamazepine. Photoparoxysmal response in EEG occurs around puberty and disappears as age advances. It usually disappears in 80% of patients treated with valproate. Adult patients with JME may not show a photoparoxysmal response. A family history of JME is seen in 50% of patients. Although JME has been extensively studied, no single gene has been identified for the syndrome. The diagnosis of JME is important in order to decide on the right antiepileptic drug (AED). Sodium valproate is the drug of choice; however, in young women of childbearing age, levetiracetam or lamotrigine should be considered as the first option as valproate is associated with neural tube defects and decreased IQ in children of mothers exposed to valproate. Patients usually have a good response to sodium valproate or levetiracetam. Lamotrigine can worsen myoclonic jerks, which can be controlled by adjunct therapy with clonazepam. The other second-line adjunct drugs, which are recommended, are topiramate and zonisamide. Patients treated with sodium channel blockers can experience worsening of seizures and myoclonic jerks, hence sodium channel blockers are to be avoided in these patients. Previous studies showed seizure remission in almost 90% of patients while on treatment, with recurrence on dose reduction or withdrawal of AEDs in over 85% of patients.[4] A recent study by Geithner et al. in 2012 followed up 31 patients for a minimum of 25 years to identify the predictors of long-term seizure outcome.[5] It was found that GTCS following bilateral myoclonic jerks, long duration of epilepsy which is uncontrolled, AED polytherapy, and photoparoxysmal response in EEG on AED withdrawal were important predictors for poor seizure outcome. Notably, six of the patients studied remained in remission following withdrawal of AEDs. Currently, consensus is that AED treatment should be continued for long term in JME patients.

Mesial Temporal Lobe Sclerosis

Mesial temporal lobe epilepsy (MTLE) is an important cause of focal-onset epilepsy in adults. It occurs due to focal neuronal loss and gliosis in the hippocampus causing MTLS. The patients develop seizure in late childhood or adolescence and may have a previous history of febrile seizures. Patients usually have an aura before the seizure, which is described as an epigastric sensation or intense fear. Some patients have gustatory or olfactory aura, while few have autonomic or psychic symptoms. Most patients have oroalimentary automatisms with a staring look. Occasionally, there may also be posturing of the contralateral upper limb. Focal seizures may progress to GTCSs. Neurological examination is otherwise normal, except for mild memory deficits. MRI of the brain shows hippocampal sclerosis while interictal EEG may show temporal spikes. Since the medial temporal lobe is deep-seated, surface EEG may be normal. Patients are usually treated with a sodium channel blocker such as carbamazepine, oxcarbazepine, lamotrigine, or lacosamide. Patients who do not respond to first-line treatment may need an add-on with a second AED with a different mechanism of action. Choice of add-on drug depends on the patient profile and comorbid conditions.

Commonly used add-on drugs are clobazam, levetiracetam, valproate, topiramate, zonisamide, and lamotrigine. Those patients, who are truly resistant to medical treatment, are candidates for surgical intervention.

SECONDARY NEW-ONSET EPILEPSY IN ADULTS

Many of the adult-onset epilepsies may be secondary to acquired insults to the brain such as infections, trauma, and stroke (Table 1). Neurocysticercosis (NCC) and neurotuberculosis are the two common infections, which can cause secondary NOEA in the Indian context. Post-traumatic and poststroke seizures are also significant. Metabolic abnormalities such as hypocalcemia, hypoglycemia, hyponatremia, drug-induced seizures, and essential oil-related seizures can be mistaken for primary NOEA if the true causative factors are not identified.

Infections

Neurocysticercosis is an infection of the central nervous system (CNS) by the larvae of *Taenia solium*. Patients present with focal onset or generalized seizures. NCC is diagnosed based on typical MRI characteristics like the presence of a scolex on neuroimaging. NCC granulomas may be mistaken for tuberculomas and patients may be treated with antitubercular drugs. There are a few key features, which help to differentiate NCC from tuberculosis (TB) granulomas which are enlisted in Table 2. Patients with NCC

Table 2: Differences between neurocysticercal and tuberculous granulomas.

Clinical features	Neurocysticercosis	Tuberculosis
Isolated seizures	Common	Associated systemic symptoms of fever, weight loss, and headache
Multiorgan involvement	Subcutaneous nodules, ocular cysticerci/cysticercal nodules in the tongue	Yes, may have tuberculosis (TB) in other organs like lung, liver, lymph node, and bone
Laboratory parameters	Normal	Raised ESR, anemia
MRI sequences	Neurocysticercosis (Fig. 1)	Caseating TB granuloma (Figs. 2A to C)
T2-weighted image	• Cystic contents appear hyperintense • Hypointense wall is present	Hypointense lesion with hyperintense center
T2-FLAIR-weighted image	Scolex, if visible is diagnostic. Complete or partial inversion (hypointense content with hyperintense wall)	No inversion
T1-FLAIR-weighted image	• Hypointense content • Scolex may be seen	Iso- to hypointense lesion with more hypointense center
Diffusion-weighted image	Scolex or degenerating cyst may show restriction	Diffusion restriction, if necrotic center is present
Postcontrast T1-weighted image	• *Ring enhancement*: Single or coalescent lesions • Usually thin-walled lesion	• Ring enhancement with hypointense center • Thick-walled conglomerate lesions may be seen

(ESR: erythrocyte sedimentation rate; FLAIR: fluid-attenuated inversion recovery)

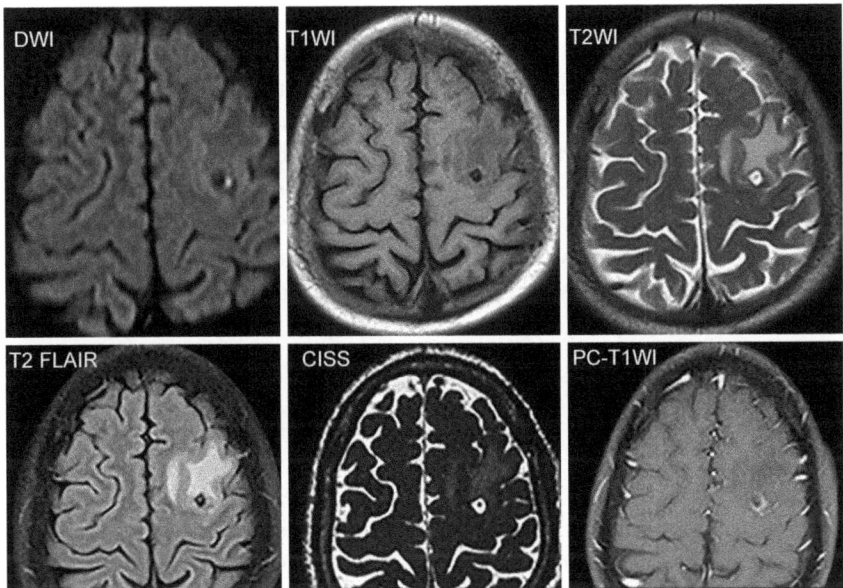

Fig. 1: Neurocysticercosis in the left posterior frontal region showing scolex on DWI, CISS and FLAIR sequences. Tiny ring enhancement is noted with perilesional edema.

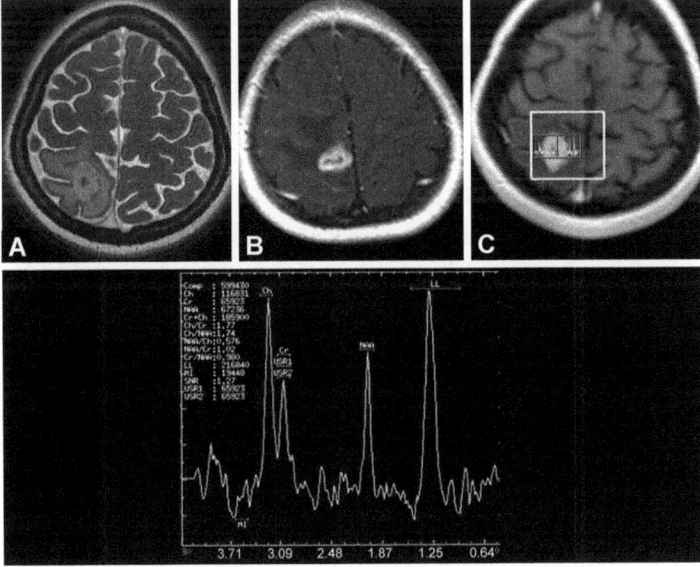

Figs. 2A to C: Right parietal tuberculoma: (A) T2WI showing well-defined oval shaped lesion noted with central T2 shortening and perilesional edema; (B) Post contrast T1WI showing irregular thick-walled ring enhancing lesion; (C) MR Spectroscopy is showing large lipid-lactate peak. Tall choline peak is also common in caseating tuberculomas with solid center. However, Cho: Cr <2 unlike high grade neoplastic lesions where this ratio is >2.

are treated with short course of steroids along with albendazole 15 mg/kg/day in two divided doses for 2–4 weeks. AED should be continued for

6 months after the radiographic resolution of the active infection. Notably, calcified granulomas can appear as ring-enhancing lesions due to seizure activity. They do not require any specific treatment and should be treated with AEDs only. Seizures due to tuberculosis are treated with AEDs like levetiracetam, which have no significant hepatotoxicity. Seizures can often occur during acute herpes simplex encephalitis and sometimes as sequelae. Human immunodeficiency virus (HIV) and neurosyphilis can also cause chronic infection in the CNS and can manifest with seizures. Though HIV per se can cause seizures, one must rule out opportunistic infections such as toxoplasmosis, TB, or cryptococcal meningitis.

Structural

Poststroke Seizures

There is an increased risk for seizures after ischemic stroke and intracranial bleed. Early-onset seizures occur within 2 weeks of stroke and are due to biochemical disruption. They carry only 20% risk of recurrence. Remote symptomatic seizures due to gliosis occur at variable periods of weeks to years after stroke and have almost 60% chance of recurrence. These patients are treated as poststroke epilepsy.[6] However, there is no role for prophylactic antiepileptics for seizure prevention in ischemic strokes. In patients with cerebral venous thrombosis, there is a high risk of seizure if patients have parenchymal hemorrhagic lesions. These patients are treated with any of the standard AEDs.

Post-traumatic

Head trauma patients have a higher risk of seizures. Post-traumatic seizures occurring within 1 week of insult to the brain are considered to be acute symptomatic seizures and do not need long-term AED therapy. Post-traumatic epilepsy (PTE) is characterized by unprovoked seizures that occur after 1 week of traumatic brain injury. The risk factors for PTE include intracranial hemorrhage and presence of depressed skull fracture, which is consistent with severe traumatic brain injury. The risk remains high even after a decade of trauma and patients require AEDs for a long time.

Tumors

Patients with brain tumors and metastatic lesions to the brain can manifest focal-onset seizures and are easily diagnosed based on MRI. In primary brain tumors, 30–70% of cases develop epilepsy. Epilepsy is more often seen in low-grade tumors such as astrocytoma, oligodendroglioma, and meningioma when compared to highly cellular tumors like malignant gliomas.[7] Thus, patients presenting with epilepsy due to brain tumors have a good prognosis since they have a favorable histology. The tumors are identified earlier due to seizures before they cause mass effect and neurological deficits. These tumors also have a superficial cortical location, which makes them amenable to complete resection. However, the seizures may be difficult to control and are often pharmacoresistant. Since the use of AEDs has not been found to reduce the rate of epileptogenesis, they are not recommended as prophylaxis in brain tumor patients without seizures.

Autoimmune Encephalitis

Autoimmune encephalitis is now recognized as an important cause of epilepsy. Autoimmune etiology should be suspected when a patient has a subacute onset of recurrent seizures with memory impairment, behavioral changes, and movement disorders. Patients with autoimmune encephalitis should be screened for possible malignancy. Patients respond to immunomodulation with high-dose steroids or intravenous (IV) immunoglobulin. Patients may need long-term immunosuppression with steroids or rituximab. Another condition seen in older adults is Steroid-Responsive Encephalopathy associated with Autoimmune Thyroiditis (SREAT), earlier referred to as Hashimoto's encephalopathy. Patients present with encephalopathy, seizures, or focal deficits with normal MRI and high anti-thyroid peroxidase (anti-TPO) titers, and usually respond well to steroids. Systemic lupus erythematosus can affect the CNS causing neuropsychiatric manifestations and seizures. Demyelinating disorders of the CNS like multiple sclerosis and neuromyelitis optica do not commonly present with seizures. However, there is a rare subset of myelin oligodendrocyte glycoprotein (MOG) antibody-positive patients who present with focal cortical encephalitis. These patients can have seizures with headache or behavioral changes. They respond well to steroids.

Essential Oil-related Seizures

Essential oil-related seizures are under recognized. Various plant-derived essential oils have been known for over a century to have epileptogenic properties. A survey of the literature shows essential oils of 12 plants—eucalyptus, camphor, fennel, hyssop, pennyroyal, rosemary, sage, savin, tansy, thuja, turpentine, and wormwood to be powerful convulsants.[8] Eucalyptus and camphor contain the monoterpene, 1,8-cineole, which acts like pentylenetetrazole and can precipitate seizures by CNS stimulant action.[9] Inhalation of essential oils has the fastest onset of action compared to topical application or ingestion. In a recent prospective observational study from Bengaluru, 37 patients with essential oil-related seizures were identified.[10] Of the 37 patients, 16 had essential oil-induced seizures (EOIS) and 21 had essential oil-provoked seizures (EOPS). Modes of exposure were local, inhalation, and ingestion. Most patients had GTCS and the fastest onset was noticed after inhalation of essential oils. Majority of patients with essential oil-related seizures did not have recurrence of seizures after stopping the essential oil usage.

INVESTIGATIONS

Investigations are necessary in most adult-onset epilepsy. MRI of brain is invaluable in excluding a structural cause. EEG is needed to diagnose epileptic syndromes such as JME and MTLS. A complete biochemical evaluation including blood sugar, renal function tests, liver function test, serum sodium, calcium, and magnesium should be checked. In diabetic patients, frequent monitoring of sugars should be done to exclude hypoglycemia. In patients with other systemic symptoms, HIV, venereal disease research laboratory (VDRL), and antinuclear antibody (ANA) must be tested. In subacute-onset epilepsy of presumed autoimmune or paraneoplastic etiology, a panel of autoimmune and paraneoplastic antibodies should be tested in standardized laboratories. A practical approach to patients presenting with new-onset epilepsy is elucidated in Flowchart 1.

CONCLUSION

New-onset epilepsy in adults has many causes varying from idiopathic/genetic, infectious, metabolic, autoimmune, stroke, trauma, and tumors. A detailed history remains the cornerstone for reaching a correct diagnosis of a seizure/epilepsy. All triggering factors for seizure like drugs and essential oil exposure must be thoroughly checked for and excluded before labeling a seizure as unprovoked/idiopathic. Patients with epilepsy due to structural causes may require long-term AEDs. Patients should be counseled about compliance to treatment. If diagnosed and treated correctly, epilepsy can be well-controlled in most patients.

ACKNOWLEDGMENT

We thank Dr Sharath Kumar GG, Consultant Neuroradiologist (Apollo and St John's Hospitals, Bengaluru) for the MR images of cysticercosis and tuberculoma and for his inputs regarding MRI features differentiating cysticercosis and tuberculosis.

Flowchart 1: Practical approach.

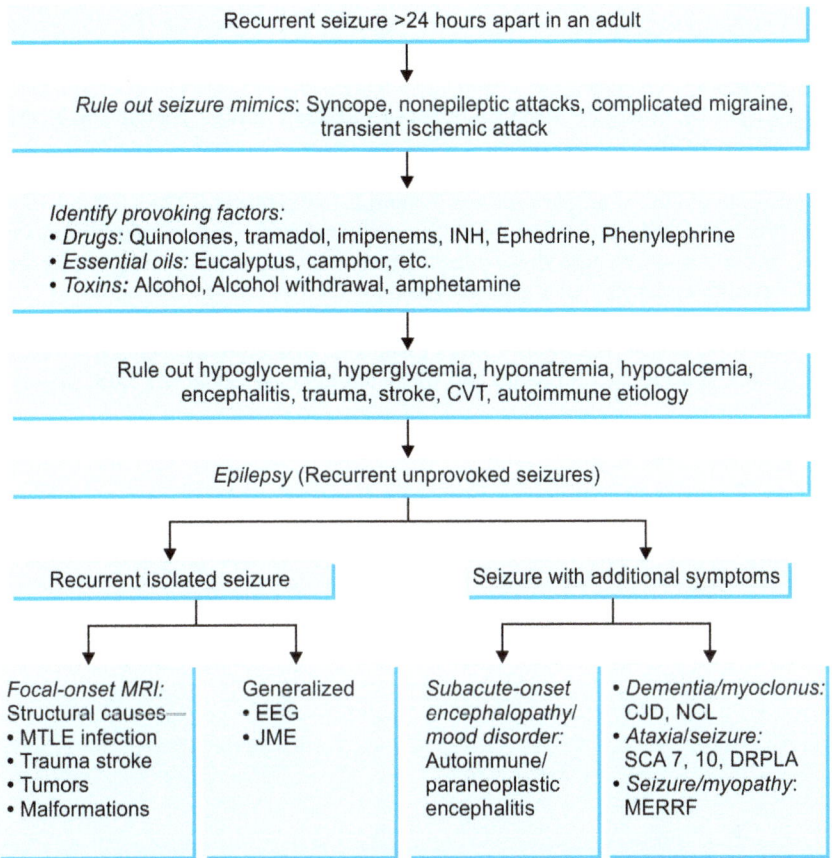

(CJD: Creutzfeldt–Jakob disease; CVT: cerebral venous thrombosis; DRPLA: dentatorubral-pallidoluysian atrophy; EEG: electroencephalogram; INH: isoniazid; JME: juvenile myoclonic epilepsy; MERRF: myoclonic epilepsy with ragged red fibers; MTLE: mesial temporal lobe epilepsy; NCL: neuronal ceroid lipofuscinosis; SCA: spinocerebellar ataxia)

REFERENCES

1. Fisher RS, Acevedo C, Arzimanoglou A, et al. ILAE Official Report: a practical clinical definition of epilepsy. Epilepsia. 2014;55(4):475-82.
2. Marini C, King MA, Archer JS, et al. Idiopathic generalised epilepsy of adult onset: clinical syndromes and genetics. J Neurol Neurosurg Psychiatry. 2003;74(2):192-6.
3. Vijai J, Cherian PJ, Sylaja PN, et al. Clinical characteristics of a South Indian cohort of juvenile myoclonic epilepsy probands. Seizure. 2003;12:490-6.
4. Janz D. Epilepsy with impulsive petit mal (Juvenile Myoclonic Epilepsy). Acta Neurol Scand. 1985;72(5):449-59.

5. Geithner J, Schneider F, Wang Z, et al. Predictors for long-term seizure outcome in juvenile myoclonic epilepsy: 25-63 years of follow-up. Epilepsia. 2012;53(8):1379-86.
6. Camilo O, Goldstein LB. Seizures and epilepsy after ischemic stroke. Stroke. 2004;35(7):1769-75.
7. Englot DJ, Chang EF, Vecht CJ. Epilepsy and brain tumors. Handb Clin Neurol. 2016;134:267-85.
8. Burkhard PR, Burkhardt K, Haenggeli CA, et al. Plant-induced seizures: reappearance of an old problem. J Neurol. 1999;246(8):667-70.
9. Mathew T, Kamath V, Kumar RS, et al. Eucalyptus oil inhalation-induced seizure: a novel, underrecognized, preventable cause of acute symptomatic seizure. Epilepsia Open. 2017;2(3):350-4.
10. Mathew T, Kamath V, Jadav R, et al. Essential Oil-induced (EOIS) and Provoked Seizures (EOPS)—A Multicentric Prospective Observational Study from South India. Indonesia: 12th Asian and Oceanian Epilepsy Congress; 2018.

5
Epilepsy in Elderly

Satishchandra P, Viswanathan LG, Sanjib Sinha

INTRODUCTION

Studies that have looked into the epidemiology of seizures suggest that increased life expectancy occurs more frequently after 60 years of age.[1,2] The clinical features, etiology, and the psychosocial impact of epilepsy are different in elderly population. Furthermore, elderly persons with epilepsy have about 3 times increased mortality compared to the healthy population. Also, other common diseases may present like seizures (Box 1).

Pharmacodynamics and pharmacokinetics of antiepileptic drugs (AEDs) in this age group are also distinctive.

This chapter deliberates the epidemiology, etiology, diagnosis, and treatment options of epilepsy, including status epilepticus (SE) in the elderly.

Box 1: Differential diagnoses of seizures in elderly people.

Neurological:
- Transient ischemic attack
- Narcolepsy
- Restless legs syndrome (sensory seizures)
- Postural instability

Cardiovascular:
- Vasovagal syncope
- Orthostatic hypotension
- Cardiac arrhythmias
- Structural heart disease
- Carotid sinus syndrome

Endocrine/metabolic:
- Hypo-/hyperglycemia
- Hypo-/hypernatremia
- Abnormalities in calcium/phosphorus metabolism
- Thyrotoxicosis

Sleep disorders:
- Sleep apnea
- Hypnic jerks
- Rapid eye movement (REM) behavior

Psychological:
- Nonepileptic psychogenic seizures

EPIDEMIOLOGY, CLASSIFICATION, AND ETIOLOGY

Population-based studies have indicated a higher incidence of seizures among elderly patients and increasing age itself might be a risk factor.[3] In USA, the annual incidence of seizures is almost 100/100,000 persons >60 years of age.[4] Whereas in the UK, >11 million elderly individuals live, and among them at least 1% might have epilepsy.[1]

In most geriatric patients, seizures are symptomatic. Acute symptomatic seizures happen in the setting of an acute brain injury or during metabolic derangement.[1,5,6] Provoked seizures are related to stroke, neuroinfections, hyper-/hypoglycemia, dyselectrolytemia, uremia, and alcohol withdrawal. Almost a third of acute seizures among older subjects manifest as SE, with a mortality of about 40%. The annual incidence of epilepsy increases with time from 90/100,000 in people between 65 years and 69 years to >150/100,000 for those over 80 years.[7] In India, the prevalence and incidence are higher in the first 30 years and unlike elsewhere, it is lower in older age. Results from a meta-analysis showed that prevalence rate was more in 10–19 years age group (0.89%), then continued to decrease with age, viz. 0.21% among >50 years.[8] In the Bangalore Urban and Rural Neuro epidemiological (BURN) survey, 8.8/1,000 population were the prevalence rate, with twice the rate in rural population than in urban regions.[9] Among those >60 years of age, the rural and urban prevalence were 3.5/1,000 and 6.4/1,000 population, respectively. From Kerala, Radhakrishnan et al. in 2000 reported a lesser prevalence rate of epilepsy among elderly (2.8/1,000) compared to overall cohort (4.93/1,000).[10]

Epilepsies and epileptic syndromes might be classified as localization related (focal) or generalized, based on clinical and electroencephalogram (EEG) findings.[6] A generalized epilepsy or epileptic syndrome might be due to involvement of both the cerebral hemispheres symmetrically at seizure onset. In focal epilepsy, seizures arise in a specific cortical region, thereby causing specific clinical manifestations, and might be associated with or without impaired awareness.

PROVOKED SEIZURES

The single most common cause of provoked seizures among elderly people is acute stroke. Eight percent of them might develop seizures within 14 days of hemorrhagic stroke, while 5% develop following an ischemic stroke. Metabolic and electrolyte disturbances such as hypoglycemia, hyperglycemia, uremia, hyponatremia, hypocalcemia, hypothyroidism, chest infections, urinary tract infection (UTI), and liver failure could precipitate seizures. Seizures secondary to acute cerebral infections occur less commonly in developed world than in developing ones. Some of the medications commonly used by elderly patients might precipitate ictus, e.g. theophylline, antidepressants, levodopa, neuroleptics, antibiotics, Ginkgo biloba, and thiazides.

FIRST UNPROVOKED SEIZURE AND EPILEPSY

Elderly individuals manifesting with initial acute symptomatic seizure are more likely to develop epilepsy than younger patients. Chronic infarcts (nonlacunar) are a common underlying cause, accounting for 30–40% of patients. Subclinical cerebral ischemia could be responsible for epilepsy in a few. Dementias including Alzheimer's disease, etc. might be associated with 5–10 times higher risk of epilepsy, especially in the advanced stage. Brain tumors and traumatic brain injury (TBI) are lesser common causes of seizures in this age group.[5,11,12]

DIAGNOSTIC EVALUATION

The approach to investigating a patient with epilepsy has been covered elsewhere in this book. Similar principles used in adults may be extrapolated to the elderly population. Review of current drugs, including over-the-counter (OTC) medications, is must, because some of them may lower the seizure threshold. Laboratory tests should include: hemogram, liver and renal function tests, serum electrolytes and sugar, X-ray of chest, and an electrocardiogram (ECG). When clinically indicated, serum AED concentrations and toxicology screen may be performed. Cardiac workup is essential in those with syncope, or transient ischemic attack (TIA). MRI is the investigation of choice and is better than CT scan in detecting abnormalities. Age-related changes, including diffuse brain atrophy, periventricular hyperintensities due to hypertension, and atherosclerosis, are common in this age group and should be interpreted with caution as the cause of seizures.[13] Cerebrospinal fluid (CSF) examination may be done if meningitis is considered, or is immunocompromised.

Epilepsy among the elderly variably affects the functional status and quality-of-life (QoL). The aim of treatment should be to adequately control seizures and improve QoL. Preferably, treatment with the least effective dosage with a single drug is advisable. Most AEDs can cause excessive sleep and worsen cognition. Nevertheless, the second-generation AEDs might have certain advantages over first-generation AEDs, but affordability may be a limiting factor for populations in developing nations. The favored AEDs among elderly patients comprise levetiracetam (LVM), gabapentin, lamotrigine, and valproic acid.

ANTIEPILEPTIC DRUG SELECTION

Management of acute seizures requires AEDs (duration variable, from weeks to months) whereas single seizure due to reversible cause (e.g. hypoglycemia) might not require long-term AEDs. Whether the first seizure requires treatment is controversial. Patients having onset with SE, recurrent seizures, or a structural pathology for seizures might require AEDs. The ideal AED is one with one or twice daily dosage, less price, favorable side effect profile, and drug interactions and availability in a parenteral form.

The decision to select AEDs in the elderly requires evidence, experience, and often cost, which becomes a limiting factor. The older AEDs, such as carbamazepine (CBZ), phenytoin, valproic acid, are less expensive than the newer drugs and are often considered for the treatment of seizures in the elderly.

ANTIEPILEPTIC MEDICATIONS

The older generation AEDs, except for ethosuximide, are effective against focal seizures with/without generalization. CBZ may be superior for control of focal seizures compared to sodium valproate; however, there are no trials involving elderly subjects to support this. Phenobarbitone is not usually recommended in elderly people due to the sedation. With phenytoin, the pharmacokinetics changes from first to zero order at convention dosages, hence blood levels may be performed periodically to avoid toxicity. Hyponatremia due to CBZ occurs more commonly later in life and diligent monitoring is advisable. Phenytoin, phenobarbitone, and CBZ can cause drug-drug interactions with antiarrhythmic, warfarin, steroids, theophylline, cytotoxics, antidepressants, and antibiotics. Enzyme induction increases vitamin D metabolism, which may lead to deficiency states and poor bone health.

Consequently, calcium and vitamin D supplements may be prescribed and periodic bone density measurements for elderly subjects at risk for osteoporosis, viz. prolonged treatment, multiple medications, or prolonged nonambulation is a good practice point.[14,15]

None of the newer AEDs is superior to the conventional AEDs for the management of new-onset diagnosed partial seizures and generalized tonic-clonic seizure (GTCS), though lamotrigine and oxcarbazepine have reported better tolerability, and hence better outcome. Newer AEDs as first-line medication in the older age include gabapentin, lamotrigine, and oxcarbazepine. The newer AEDs have better side effect profiles and less drug interactions than the conventional AEDs.[16,17]

It is recommended to start low and go slow with monotherapy, ideally with a drug, which causes least interactions with other drugs co-prescribed and one that has a favorable adverse effect profile. The VA cooperative study on the effects of age on epilepsy and its treatment showed that in contrast with younger age group,[18] elderly subjects respond to AEDs better, but might suffer from more adverse reactions. Estimation of the unbound drug concentration could be beneficial, particularly when the response is inappropriate.

STATUS EPILEPTICUS AMONG ELDERLY

Status epilepticus (SE) is a medical emergency, which requires aggressive and urgent treatment, especially for elderly individuals in whom comorbid conditions may increase the severity of consequences in SE.[12] There is no established protocol for SE management in elderly patients and recommendations for management of SE in elderly subjects are similar to those in young adults. The therapeutic approach requires special attention because physiological changes with age and increased use of polypharmacy cause complex pharmacokinetics in the elderly than in younger individuals (Box 2). Among the newer AEDs, LVM has good pharmacokinetic profile and fewer drug interactions and is well-tolerated in critically ill elderly subjects.[17,18] According to a study done by Berning et al. in 2009, LVM is effective in the treatment of SE, and might be a good practical alternative to multimorbid elderly patients who need parenteral AED. Injectable lacosamide is a promising AED, which seems to have a good pharmacokinetics and might turn to be useful among elderly subjects with SE.

Box 2: Pharmacological considerations in elderly people.

Pharmacokinetic
Reduction in:
- Protein binding
- Hepatic metabolism
- Enzyme inducibility
- Renal elimination

Pharmacodynamic
Alterations in:
- Brain neurotransmitters
- Receptor function
- Autonomic pharmacology
- Homeostatic mechanisms

Tolerability
Greater risk of:
- Altered kinetics and dynamics
- Polypharmacy and interactions
- Idiosyncratic reactions
- Physical and psychiatric comorbidities

CONCLUSION

Epilepsy has bimodal distribution; first peak is during the 1st and 2nd decades and second peak is seen in the elderly above the age of 60 years. With recommended treatment, seizures can be well-controlled in most elderly people with epilepsy. While choosing an AED, one needs to consider adverse effects and drug-drug interactions of AEDs as these patients may be on many drugs for various comorbidities. Randomized controlled trials (RCTs) show that lamotrigine and gabapentin are preferred in older individuals. The negative impact of epilepsy on physical and psychological well-being affects the QoL. The number of older subjects with epilepsy is expected to increase and poses a great burden on healthcare resources.

REFERENCES

1. Brodie MJ, Kwan P. Epilepsy in elderly people. BMJ. 2005;331(7528):1317-22.
2. DeToledo JC. Changing presentation of seizures with aging: clinical and etiological factors. Gerontology. 1999;45(6):329-35.
3. Hauser WA. Seizure disorders: the changes with age. Epilepsia. 1992;33 Suppl 4:S6-14.
4. Faught E. Epidemiology and drug treatment of epilepsy in elderly people. Drugs Aging. 1999;15(4):255-69.
5. Hauser WA, Annegers JF, Kurland LT. Incidence of epilepsy and unprovoked seizures in Rochester, Minnesota: 1935-1984. Epilepsia. 1993;34(3):453-68.
6. Proposal for revised classification of epilepsies and epileptic syndromes. Commission on Classification and Terminology of the International League Against Epilepsy. Epilepsia. 1989;30(4):389-99.
7. Wallace H, Shorvon S, Tallis R. Age-specific incidence and prevalence rates of treated epilepsy in an unselected population of 2,052,922 and age-specific fertility rates of women with epilepsy. Lancet. 1998;352(9145):1970-3.
8. Sridharan R, Murthy BN. Prevalence and pattern of epilepsy in India. Epilepsia. 1999;40(5):631-6.
9. Gourie-Devi M, Gururaj G, Satishchandra P, et al. Prevalence of neurological disorders in Bangalore, India: a community-based study with a comparison between urban and rural areas. Neuroepidemiology. 2004;23(6):261-8.
10. Radhakrishnan K, Pandian JD, Santhoshkumar T, et al. Prevalence, knowledge, attitude, and practice of epilepsy in Kerala, South India. Epilepsia. 2000;41(8):1027-35.
11. Lühdorf K, Jensen LK, Plesner AM. Etiology of seizures in the elderly. Epilepsia. 1986;27(4):458-63.
12. Sinha S, Satishchandra P, Kalband BR, et al. New-onset status epilepticus and cluster seizures in the elderly. J Clin Neurosci. 2013;20(3):423-8.
13. Sinha S, Satishchandra P, Kalband BR, et al. Neuroimaging observations in a cohort of elderly manifesting with new onset seizures: experience from a university hospital. Ann Indian Acad Neurol. 2012;15(4):273-80.
14. Krämer G. Epilepsy in the elderly: some clinical and pharmacotherapeutic aspects. Epilepsia. 2001;42 Suppl 3:55-9.
15. French JA, Kanner AM, Bautista J, et al. Efficacy and tolerability of the new antiepileptic drugs II: treatment of refractory epilepsy: report of the

Therapeutics and Technology Assessment Subcommittee and Quality Standards Subcommittee of the American Academy of Neurology and the American Epilepsy Society. Neurology. 2004;62(8):1261-73.
16. Rowan AJ, Ramsay RE, Collins JF, et al. New onset geriatric epilepsy: a randomized study of gabapentin, lamotrigine, and carbamazepine. Neurology. 2005;64(11):1868-73.
17. Ferrendelli JA, French J, Leppik I, et al. Use of levetiracetam in a population of patients aged 65 years and older: a subset analysis of the KEEPER trial. Epilepsy Behav. 2003;4(6):702-9.
18. Treiman DM, Meyers PD, Walton NY, et al. A comparison of four treatments for generalized convulsive status epilepticus. Veterans Affairs Status Epilepticus Cooperative Study Group. N Engl J Med. 1998;339(12):792-8.

6

Women, Epilepsy and Pregnancy

Agadi JB

INTRODUCTION

Menstrual irregularities, social stigma, low rates of marriage, infertility, and recurrence of seizures during pregnancy, labor, or postpartum are the problems faced by women with epilepsy. The purpose of management of epilepsy during pregnancy is to ensure that the mother remains healthy at the end of pregnancy and child birth and delivers a healthy baby. Physicians treating epilepsy during pregnancy should be aware of the efficacy as well as the teratogenic potential of the antiepileptic drugs (AEDs). Women with epilepsy (WWE) in the reproductive age group should be advised to avoid unplanned pregnancies. Women are often unfamiliar with the teratogenic risks of AEDs and their interaction with contraception.[1] Out of 2.73 million WWE in India, 1.5 million are in the reproductive age group.[2] There are conditions that cause seizures during pregnancy like metabolic derangements, eclampsia, and cerebral venous sinus thrombosis and they will not be addressed here.

EFFECT OF PREGNANCY ON EPILEPSY

Poor compliance is the main cause for recurrence of seizures in nearly one-third of WWE with pregnancy who experience exaggeration of seizures. Mental stress, hormonal imbalance, lack of sleep, and hyperemesis are some of the causes of exaggeration of seizures during the 1st trimester. Hemodilution and increased elimination with lowered serum concentration are the other contributing factors, especially for drugs like lamotrigine (LTG), levetiracetam, and oxcarbazepine.

Factors that predict the recurrence of seizures during pregnancy include polytherapy, poor seizure control in the 9-12 months prior to pregnancy. About 7-25% show improvement and 50-83% show no change in seizure frequency.[3]

EFFECT OF EPILEPSY ON PREGNANCY

Epilepsy has a significant impact on the obstetric outcome. Studies have shown increased rates for spontaneous miscarriages, antepartum hemorrhage, hypertensive disorders, and postpartum hemorrhage. There is increased incidence of induction of labor, cesarean section, preterm birth, and fetal growth restriction. Generalized tonic-clonic seizures during pregnancy can cause maternal and fetal hypoxia, acidosis, decreased fetal heart rate, miscarriages, and stillbirth. Trauma sustained during seizure can lead to premature rupture of membranes, which can lead to infection, premature labor, and even fetal death. Reemergence of seizures can be devastating with a 10-fold increase in mortality.[3] Gestational diabetes, preterm birth, stillbirth, prenatal or perinatal death, and admission to neonatal intensive care unit did not differ between women with epilepsy and those without the disorder.[4]

TERATOGENIC EFFECTS OF ANTIEPILEPTIC DRUGS

Neural tube starts forming 3 days after the missed menstrual period and closes between 3 weeks and 4 weeks. Cleft lip occurs before 5 weeks, congenital heart diseases occur before 6 weeks, and cleft palate occurs before 10 weeks. AEDs exert their most serious effects during the first 10 weeks.

Major congenital malformations (MCMs) are defined as "structural abnormalities of surgical, medical, and functional or cosmetic importance", which occur during organogenesis in the 1st trimester.[5]

Antiepileptic drug-induced cardiac malformations include Fallot's tetralogy, atrial septal defect, ventricular septal defect, patent ductus arteriosus, pulmonary atresia, and single ventricle, etc. Nervous system malformations include neural tube defects. Craniofacial defects like cleft lip and palate can occur. Esophageal atresia, congenital hypertrophic pyloric stenosis, inguinal, diaphragmatic, omphalocele, and umbilical hernias occur as gastrointestinal malformations. Renal agenesis, hydronephrosis, hypospadias, and undescended testis can occur.[6]

Midline craniofacial anomalies, ocular hypertelorism, broad epicanthic folds, short upturned nose, altered lips, low hairline, and digital and nail hypoplasia are known to occur as minor congenital malformations and do not constitute a threat to life.

Sodium valproate (VA), primidone, and carbamazepine (CBZ) are known to cause fetal AED syndrome. Fetal AED syndrome consists of midfacial hypoplasia, long upper lip, low birth weight, cleft lip and palate, and digital and nail hypoplasia.

In a study from the UK epilepsy and pregnancy registry, 4.2% of live births to women with epilepsy had major congenital malformations. It is observed that there is dose-dependent increase in the rate of congenital malformations more with polytherapy than with monotherapy. Sodium VA caused the highest rate of major congenital malformations when compared to other drugs. There was a dose-dependent increase in the risk of MCMs for

CBZ, LTG, VA, and phenobarbital (PB). For CBZ, the incidence of MCMs was 3.4% when the dosage was less than 400 mg and it rose to 8.7% when the dosage was increased to 1,000 mg/day. For phenobarbitone, the incidence of MCMs was 5.4% when the dosage was less than 150 mg/day and the incidence rose to 13.7% when the dosage was more than 150 mg/day. For LTG, the incidence was 2% when the dosage was less than 200 mg/day and the incidence rose to 4.5% when the dosage of LTG was more than 300 mg/day. For VA, the incidence of MCM was 5.6% when the dosage was less than 700 mg/day and the incidence rose to 24.2% when the dosage was more than 1,500 mg/day.[7] For topiramate monotherapy, the relative risk (RR) for oral clefts associated with doses less than 100 mg was 1.64 and for doses more than 100 mg it was 5.16 [95% confidence interval (CI) 1.94–13.73].[8]

The recurrence risk of malformation was 50% for women who had two previous children with a congenital malformation. For women whose first child had a congenital malformation, there was a 16.8% risk of having another child with a congenital malformation compared with 9.8% for women whose first child did not have a malformation.[9]

COGNITIVE TERATOGENESIS

Neurodevelopmental effects of CBZ, VA, phenytoin (DPH), and LTG have been studied in the US and UK. It was demonstrated that VA-exposed children had lower IQ at 6 years compared to the other drugs studied. When the dosage of VA was more than 1,000 mg, it negatively correlated with IQ, verbal ability, nonverbal ability, memory, and executive function. Other AEDs did not have a dose effect.[10]

From Liverpool and Manchester, the neurodevelopmental research group reported that autism spectrum disorder was the most frequent diagnosis for the VA-exposed children.[11]

Children exposed to levetiracetam in utero were superior in their language and motor development when compared to children exposed to sodium VA.[1]

MANAGEMENT STRATEGIES

It is too late to make medication adjustments when pregnancy has occurred. One should not change AED medication in an established pregnancy and risk the woman for the occurrence of seizures. Addition of AEDs exposes the fetus to the teratogenic effect of the added drug.

When pregnancy has advanced for several weeks, there is little advantage of changing the AED. It is ideal for the woman to consult the neurologist before she starts the family. The neurologist at this point of time assesses the need for AED, reconfirms the diagnosis of epilepsy, or rules out the diagnosis of epilepsy. If the patient is found to be in remission, the AEDs are withdrawn based on the general principles of AED withdrawal. The probability of recurrence of seizures during or after the tapering and stoppage of AEDs should be discussed. Juvenile myoclonic epilepsy patients are continued on medication. It is ideal to do medication adjustments prior to pregnancy. Prepregnancy blood levels of AEDs should be checked for future reference.

It is ideal to start 5 mg of folic acid daily 1-2 months prior to pregnancy.[2] The risk of having autistic traits was significantly higher at 18 months and 36 months in those children whose mothers did not take folic acid before and during early pregnancy when compared to the children of mothers who took folic acid.[12]

An abdominal ultrasound examination to screen for major congenital malformations is done at 16-18 weeks of pregnancy. At the same time, an estimation of serum alpha-fetoprotein levels is done. If found abnormal, there would be adequate time for termination of pregnancy. When the results of the ultrasound examination are inconclusive, amniocentesis and estimation of acetylcholinesterase can be done.

Blood levels of AEDs can be done during 1st, 2nd, and 3rd trimesters of pregnancy. Anticipatory increase in the dosages of drugs like LTG, levetiracetam, and oxcarbazepine can be done. Hemodilution and metabolic changes lower the levels of AEDs, especially during the 2nd and 3rd trimesters. Vitamin K 1 mg intramuscularly is administered to those children born to mothers on enzyme-inducing AEDs.

Any AED therapy is not a contraindication for breastfeeding. Mothers are advised to breastfeed their children under supervision. Mothers should nurse their babies and then take AED medication. Mothers are advised against sleep deprivation, especially those with juvenile myoclonic epilepsy.

CONTRACEPTION

The most reliable and reversible contraception for woman is intrauterine device (IUD). The American Academy of Pediatrics recommends IUD as an optional form of contraception for teenage girls on enzyme-inducing AEDs. There could be failure of combined oral contraceptive pills in women on enzyme-inducing AEDs. LTG is metabolized by hepatic glucuronidation. Enzyme-inducing AEDs induce glucuronidation pathways and decrease LTG levels by about 50%. If topiramate is used in conjunction with combined oral contraceptive pills, condom use should be encouraged. 12 mg of perampanel decreases levonorgestrel levels by 40% and patients on perampanel should be encouraged to use additional nonhormonal methods.

Insertion of a copper IUD within 5 days of intercourse provides highly effective emergency contraception as well as ongoing contraception. Two 0.75 mg levonorgestrel pills taken 12 hours apart also provide an effective means of emergency contraception. The dosage of levonorgestrel should be doubled in women taking enzyme-inducing AEDs.[1]

CATAMENIAL EPILEPSY

In catamenial epilepsy, there is increased seizure frequency at specific times of the menstrual cycle. As per Herzog, there is a twofold increase in seizure frequency during one of the three vulnerable time periods compared to seizure frequency during the rest of the menstrual cycle. In the C1 pattern, seizures occur predominantly between −3 days and +3 days of menstrual cycle. In the C2 pattern, seizures mostly occur on days +10 and +13. In the C3 pattern, seizures are most common on days +10 and +3 of the next cycle. Progesterone may be an appropriate adjunct for patients with predominantly perimenstrual seizures.[1]

Acetazolamide at daily doses of 250–500 mg has been tried to treat patients with catamenial epilepsy. It is commenced 3 days prior to menses and continued for 3–7 days. Clobazam has also been tried to treat catamenial epilepsy. Clobazam is administered 2–7 days prior to menses and continued for about 10 days.[13]

CONCLUSION

Management of epilepsy in women of childbearing age involves close interaction between the patient, neurologist, and the family. Most women can expect safe pregnancy and healthy babies. Choice of AED is dictated by the epilepsy syndrome that the WWE is suffering from. Drugs that are known to cause MCMs should be avoided in a woman in the reproductive age group. Lowest effective dose of AED in monotherapy is preferred in the 1st trimester. Preconceptionally, folic acid is advised and should be continued throughout pregnancy. Screening for MCM with serum alpha-fetoprotein and properly conducted abdominal ultrasound scan to detect MCMs is advisable around 16–18 weeks of pregnancy. Breastfeeding should be encouraged and there are no contraindications for breastfeeding while taking AEDs old or new. IUD insertion is a very effective routine and emergency contraceptive method.

REFERENCES

1. Gerard EE, Meador KJ. Managing epilepsy in women. Continuum (Minneap Minn). 2016;22(1):204-26.
2. Thomas SV. Managing epilepsy in pregnancy. J Neurol India. 2011;13(59):59-65.
3. Pennell PP. Pregnancy, epilepsy, and women's issues. Am Acad Neurol Instit. 2013;19(3):697-714.
4. Priya B, Singh N. Pregnant women with epilepsy: management issues. J Preg Child Health. 2017;2(4):342.

5. Tomson T, Battino D. Teratogenic effects of antiepileptic drugs. Lancet Neurol. 2012;11(9):803-13.
6. Begum S, Thomas SV. Women with epilepsy in reproductive age group: special issues and management strategies. J Assoc Physicians India. 2013;61(8 Suppl):48-51.
7. Patel SI, Pennell PB. Management of epilepsy during pregnancy: an update. Ther Adv Neurol Disord. 2016;9(2):118-29.
8. Hernandez-Diaz S, Huybrechts KF, Desai RJ, et al. Topiramate use early in pregnancy and the risk of oral clefts: a pregnancy cohort study. Neurology. 2018;90(4):e342-51.
9. Campbell E, Devenney E, Morrow J, et al. Recurrence risk of congenital malformations in infants exposed to antiepileptic drugs in utero. Epilepsia. 2013;54(1):165-71.
10. Meador K, Baker GA, Browning N, et al. Foetal antiepileptic drug exposure and cognitive outcomes at age 6 years (NEAD study)—a prospective observational study. Lancet Neurol. 2013;12(3):244-52.
11. Bromley R, Mawer GE, Briggs M, et al. The prevalence of neurodevelopmental disorders in children prenatally exposed to antiepileptic drugs. J Neurol Neurosurg Psychiatry. 2012;84(6):637-43.
12. Fitzgerald S. Folic acid during pregnancy found to prevent autistic traits in children of women on AED. J Neurol Today. 2018;18(3):25-7.
13. Naymee' J, Velez-Ruiz, Pennell PB. Issues for women with epilepsy. J Neurol Clin. 2016;34(2):411-25.

7
Seizures but Not Epilepsy

Srinivas HV

INTRODUCTION

Often times, a seizure is mistakenly diagnosed as "epilepsy" and the patient is prescribed antiepileptic drugs to be taken over a long period. What is more damaging is the social consequences like "stigma" of epilepsy not only for the patient but the entire family is devastated with the diagnosis of epilepsy. Besides this, the diagnosis affects several aspects of life for the patient, e.g. education, leisure activity including sports, employment, marriage, driving, etc. One should be aware of all these social consequences when a diagnosis of epilepsy is offered.

Seizure is like "fever", which can occur due to several conditions such as hyponatremia, hypocalcemia and "epilepsy" is a definitive diagnosis such as "typhoid". Epilepsy is defined as "two or more unprovoked seizures" occurring greater than 24 hours apart or one unprovoked seizure if there is greater than 60% chances of another seizure.[1] The diagnostic steps for epilepsy are as follows:[2]
- Is it a seizure?
- If yes, are seizures provoked?
- A single unprovoked seizure—epilepsy
- Two or more unprovoked seizures—epilepsy.

IS IT A SEIZURE?

The common conditions, which are mistaken for seizures, are: (a) syncope, (b) nonepileptic disorder, and (c) panic attack.
- *Syncope*: Syncope is due to global hypoxemia of the brain resulting in blurring of vision, noises becoming distant, sweating, gradually sinking to the ground, and transient unconsciousness with few myoclonic jerks. In view of transient loss of consciousness and myoclonic jerks, it is mistaken as a seizure. The differential features are mentioned in Table 1.

    Syncope can occur due to several causes and in elderly, cardiac syncope should be considered (Box 1).
- *Nonepileptic attack disorder (psychogenic seizure, hysterical seizures)*: After syncope, this is the second most common cause mistaken as "epilepsy". This is basically attention seeking disorder, which means it occurs only

Table 1: Differentiation between syncope and seizure.		
	Syncope	*Seizure*
Onset	Gradual sinking to the ground	Usually sudden, abrupt
Duration	10–30 seconds	1–3 minutes
Precipitating factor	Common (upright posture, sight of blood, and shocking news)	Rare (flashing lights, hyperventilation)
Convulsive jerks	Uncommon	Common
Lateral tongue bite	Very rare	Common
Incontinence	Uncommon	Common
Postictal confusion	Rare (e.g. wakes up on the same spot)	Common (e.g. wakes up in different place)

Box 1: Common types of syncope.
- *Vasovagal*: Psychogenic, micturition syncope, and cough syncope
- *Cardiogenic*: Stokes-Adams syndrome, tachy-, and bradyarrhythmia
- *Orthostatic*: Diabetes, Parkinson's disease, and primary dysautonomia.

in presence of people and never occurs during sleep or when alone. The seizure is bizarre and very prolonged in duration, may be associated with heavy breathing and vocalization (Table 2). Characteristically, the eyes are closed and resists eye opening, while in epilepsy eyes are open.
- *Panic attacks*: Panic attacks, as the name implies, are due to sudden fear with symptoms of sympathetic overactivity such as tremors, palpitation, sweating, and at times are associated with hyperventilation.

IS THE SEIZURE PROVOKED?

Cerebral cortical mantle is susceptible for a variety of conditions, which can provoke a seizure. It could broadly be divided into: (a) systemic causes and (b) structural causes (Box 2).
- *Systemic causes*: Here the provoking factor is due to extracerebral causes without any structural changes in the cerebral cortex. A number of general medical conditions commonly encountered in clinical practice may present to casualty with generalized seizures, e.g. hypoglycemia, hyponatremia, etc.
- *Structural causes*: The provoking factor of direct involvement of the brain, e.g. encephalitis, due to a variety of viruses (Japanese encephalitis, herpes simplex). The importance of diagnosing a provoked seizures is, it is not epilepsy and, hence the antiepileptic drugs are stopped at the time of discharge of the patient, in metabolic disorders. Provoked seizures due to structural damage to the brain require continuation of antiepileptic drugs for a period of 3 months from the time of discharge of the patient and at 3 months follow-up, if there are no further seizures, one can withdraw the antiepileptic drugs.

Table 2: Differentiation between nonepileptic attack disorder (NEAD) and epilepsy.		
Nonepileptic attack disorder		*Epilepsy*
Age	Common in young	Any age
Gender	Common in women	Any gender
Duration	Often prolonged, occasionally hours	1–3 minutes
Trigger	Anger, stress	Unusual
Consciousness	Retained	Unconscious
Eyes	Closed/shut tightly	Open
Resisting eye opening and eye contact	Common	Absent
Pelvic thrusting, back arching, and erratic movements	Common	Rare
Response to sprinkling of water on face	Yes	No
Tongue bite	Rare	Common
Incontinence	Rare	Common
Postictal confusion	Rare	Common
Attack pattern	Variable	Stereotyped

Box 2: Provoked seizure: Common causes.

Systemic causes:
- Febrile seizures, alcohol withdrawal
- Metabolic encephalopathies (hypoglycemia, hyponatremia, hypocalcemia, and renal/hepatic encephalopathy)
- *Drugs*: Quinolones, ephedrine, and phenylephrine.

Structural causes:
- Viral encephalitis, bacterial meningitis, and head injury
- Stroke, cortical developmental, and anomalies.

A SINGLE UNPROVOKED GENUINE SEIZURE—IS IT EPILEPSY?

To treat or not to treat single unprovoked seizure is debatable.[3,4] However, if there is a provoking mechanism, one should consider to start antiepileptic drugs. If there is no provoking mechanism, e.g. structural brain damage, there is no need to start antiepileptic drugs.

Finally when there are Two or More Unprovoked Seizures—Epilepsy to be Diagnosed

It should be remembered that one should be certain of the diagnosis of epilepsy before mentioning it to the patient, because it is not only a medical problem of continuing antiepileptic drugs but the social implications. I think it is very important to remember the stigma attached to epilepsy and when one is in doubt of diagnosis, seek a second opinion or wait for a definite diagnosis.

REFERENCES

1. Fisher RS, Acevedo C, Arzimanoglou A, et al. ILAE official report: a practical clinical definition of epilepsy. Epilepsia. 2014;55(4):475-82.
2. Srinivas HV. Manual of Epilepsy-Medical Management and Social Aspects. Jaypee Brothers Medical Publishers, New Delhi; 2016.
3. Jacobs CS, Lee JW. Immediate vs delayed treatment of first unprovoked seizure: To treat, or not to treat? Neurology. 2018;91(15):684-5.
4. Krumholz A, Wiebe S, Gronseth GS, et al. Evidence-based guideline: Management of an unprovoked first seizure in adults: Report of the Guideline Development Subcommittee of the American Academy of Neurology and the American Epilepsy Society. Neurology. 2015;84(16):1705-13.

8

Epilepsy and Psychiatric Aspects

Kalyanasundaram S, Johnson Pradeep R

INTRODUCTION

Epilepsy is a chronic neurological disorder and affects around 50 million individuals worldwide. The prevalence of epilepsy, which was self-reported, was 70% and is the greatest contributor to disability-adjusted life years in neurology. It has a serious impact not only on the individual but also on the family and society. It has been reported that at least one-third of patients with active epilepsy suffer from significant impairment of emotional well-being.[1] It has long been associated with psychiatric conditions, which adds to the misery of the patients. Early recognition and management of psychiatric comorbidities in epilepsy can lead to enhanced quality of life.

DEPRESSION AND ANXIETY DISORDERS IN PEOPLE WITH EPILEPSY

"Melancholics ordinarily become epileptics, and epileptics, melancholics: what determines the preference is the direction that the malady takes; if it bears upon the body, epilepsy, if upon the intelligence, melancholy"

—**Hippocrates 400 BC**

INTRODUCTION

Depression and anxiety disorders are common psychiatric comorbid disorders in epilepsy and have been associated with suicide, suicidal ideation, stigmatization, and reduced quality of life in people with epilepsy (PWE).

EPIDEMIOLOGY

Depression and anxiety disorders have been found in high percentage in PWE compared to the general population. The epidemiology of depression in epilepsy varies depending on the diagnostic criteria, applied measures, surveyed populations, and time frames. The overall prevalence of depression in PWE is 23.1%, while for recurrent seizures it is 20–55% and in controlled epilepsy, it ranges from 3% to 9%. The overall prevalence of anxiety disorders ranges from 11% to 25%.[2]

CLINICAL FEATURES

The clinical features have a temporal relationship with seizures. Peri-ictal depressive symptoms can be subclassified as preictal, postictal, and ictal and have a temporal relationship with seizures, whereas interictal depressive symptoms do not have a temporal relationship. The most common preictal symptom of depression is low mood; it can occur several days or hours before the seizure and may become more intense 24 hours before the seizure. Postictal depressive symptoms may not occur on the same day but can occur up to 5 days later. Postictal depressive symptoms included poor frustration tolerance, loss of interest or pleasure, helplessness, irritability, feelings of low self-esteem, feelings of guilt, crying bouts, and hopelessness (state of despair). However, ictal depressive symptoms are usually of short duration and repetitive. Some of the symptoms seen in ictal depressive symptoms are loss of interest in pleasurable activities, guilt, and suicidal ideation. The depressive symptoms in 71% of PWE do not meet the criteria for a depressive episode according to the Diagnostic and Statistical Manual of Mental Disorders-IV (DSM-IV) because they were intermittently interrupted by symptom-free periods lasting from 1 day to several days. Hence, this pattern of depression may be referred to as a dysthymic disorder (chronic low mood) associated with epilepsy.

Anxiety disorders can also be classified based on the temporal relationship between symptoms and seizures. Preictal anxiety symptoms usually occur within few hours to several days before the seizure. Postictal fear mostly occurs after a seizure and usually lasts for up to 7 days. Anxiety symptoms, which present during the auras (a sensation perceived by a patient that precedes a condition affecting the brain), include nervousness, fear, anger, and irritability. Ictal fear is of sudden onset and brief duration. Seizures from anteromedial and cingulate gyrus usually cause fear and ictal fear is closely associated with temporal lobe epilepsy (TLE) (strongly with medial TLE).

ETIOLOGIES

Psychological

Learned helplessness and chronic stress exposure correspond to depression in PWE. Exposure to recurrent seizures is viewed as unpredictable, uncontrollable, and highly aversive or even life-threatening events. PWE showed reduced belief in personal control regarding health compared with their peers; this is consistent with the concept of loss of control.

Neurobiological Factors

Temporal lobe epilepsy patients are more prone to developing depression, but it is not confirmative. Overall, patients with complex partial seizures or those with mesial temporal sclerosis are more likely to have symptoms of depression.

Sheline et al. found bilateral smaller hippocampal volumes in 10 patients with a history of major depression in remission, when compared with hippocampal volumes of 10 age, sex, and height-matched healthy subjects.[3] Hippocampal volumes are inversely correlated with the duration of the disease, suggesting that patients with a chronic and active disease were more likely to have hippocampal atrophy. Studies later suggested the importance of temporolimbic structures in mood disorders.

ROLE OF ANTIEPILEPTIC DRUGS

Antiepileptic drugs (AEDs) can be generally divided into those with positive effects on mood and those with negative effects. Those with positive effect have mood stabilizing and antianxiety effects and are used in the management of withdrawal syndromes (divalproate, carbamazepine). AEDs, which act on the benzodiazepine-gamma-aminobutyric acid (GABA) receptor complex (barbiturates, topiramate, and vigabatrin), have been associated with occurrence of depressive symptoms in patients with epilepsy. Other AEDs have low incidence of depression (less than 1%).

In anxiety disorders, amygdala and hippocampus play a key role in the pathophysiology. Orbitofrontal cortex, insula, and cingulate gyrus have been implicated in the central mediation of anxiety. The GABA-A receptors, serotonin, and modulation of calcium channels also play a significant role in the pathophysiology of anxiety.

SCREENING FOR DEPRESSION

The Neurological Disorders Depression Inventory for Epilepsy (NDDI-E) is one of the most popular screening tests for depression in PWE. It is a brief six-item questionnaire that was developed and validated in the US. This questionnaire takes less than 3 minutes to complete and a cut-off score of 15 is suggestive of a major depressive episode. The Patient Health Questionnaire-2 (PHQ-2) has been validated with the above scale and Mini-International Neuropsychiatric Interview-Plus (MINI-Plus) can be used in a busy outpatient department (OPD).[4]

TREATMENT STRATEGIES FOR DEPRESSION AND ANXIETY DISORDERS IN EPILEPSY

A very important aspect in the treatment of depression and anxiety in epilepsy is identification of the same in PWE. Neurologists or physicians can manage mild-to-moderate comorbid depression but referral to psychiatrist is suggested in severe and difficult-to-treat depression, or if the patient is acutely suicidal or having psychotic symptoms. It is very vital to first optimize seizure control and minimize unwanted AED-related side effects.

Another important strategy is improving seizure control with medications or surgery. Eventhough medications are important in the treatment of depression and anxiety disorders, current guidelines suggest the use of psychotherapy as a first line of treatment. Of all the different psychotherapies, cognitive behavioral therapy (CBT) and mindfulness-based CBT such as acceptance and commitment therapy (ACT) have been associated with significant improvements on outcome measures of depression and anxiety symptoms. Significant improvement was seen on the quality of life and the effect was sustained for at least 6 months. CBT-based interventions are helpful in the prevention of major depressive episodes and suicidal tendency in patients with epilepsy.

A general recommendation for pharmacotherapy includes use of selective serotonin reuptake inhibitors (SSRIs) (e.g. escitalopram, sertraline, and fluoxetine) and selective serotonin-norepinephrine reuptake inhibitors (SNRIs) (e.g. venlafaxine, duloxetine) as first-line agents. Use of tricyclic or tetracyclic antidepressants and norepinephrine-dopamine reuptake inhibitors (NDRIs) should be avoided in the first instance. Noradrenergic and specific serotonergic antidepressants (NaSSAs) are safe in epilepsy as well. The role of benzodiazepines is important in patients with excessive anxiety symptoms in the initial stages of treatment. One must remember that it should be used with caution and for short duration of 4–6 weeks only. It is important to closely monitor patients receiving antidepressant drug therapy, especially during titration or withdrawal.[5]

PSYCHOSIS IN PERSONS WITH EPILEPSY

EPIDEMIOLOGY

The pooled estimate of prevalence of psychosis in epilepsy was 5.6%. The prevalence was estimated as 7% in TLE, 5.2% in interictal psychosis, and 2% in postictal psychosis. The overall odds ratio for risk of psychosis was 7.8 in PWE. Psychosis in epilepsy can be categorized based on the seizures or the treatment.

Ictal Psychosis

Ictal psychosis (IP) is rare and presents as a combination of cognitive, affective, and hallucinatory symptoms of partial epilepsy to produce a psychotic state. The most common symptoms include visual or auditory illusions (misinterpreted perception of a sensory experience) and hallucinations (a perception such as an image, touch, taste, sound, or smell) that seem real but do not really exist, combined with mood changes, such as agitation, fear, or paranoia. The other symptoms of partial epilepsy include depersonalization (an "as if" experience where a person feels detached or disconnected from his or her personal identity or self), derealization (an "as if" experience of the external world where they feel that it is unreal), autoscopy (visual hallucination of an image of one's body), out of body experience, or a sense of "someone behind".

Ictal psychosis is usually localized to the temporal lobe with activation of limbic and neocortical temporal areas. Prolonged IP states are rare and may occur as a nonconvulsive status epilepticus with simple or complex partial or absence seizures.

Postictal Psychosis

Postictal psychosis (PIP) can occur in 2-7.8% of PWE. It is characterized by hallucinations (false perceptions without any stimulus), delusions (a false belief that is held with strong conviction even in the presence of evidence to the contrary), and/or gross abnormalities of behavior or affect up to 7 days after a seizure. It usually occurs in those with more than 10 years of seizures and is common in both right and left TLE. As the frequency of PIP increases, the chances of developing chronic interictal psychosis also increase.

The diagnostic criteria include: (1) episode of psychosis within 1 week after a seizure(s); (2) psychosis for more than 15 hours and less than 3 months; (3) delusions, hallucinations in clear consciousness, unexpected or disorganized behavior, formal thought disorder (disorganized thinking as evidenced by disorganized speech), or mood changes; and (4) no evidence of AED toxicity, nonconvulsive status epilepticus, recent head trauma, alcohol, or drug intoxication or withdrawal, and prior chronic psychotic disorder.

The symptoms are predominantly characterized by mood abnormalities than delusions of reference, false perception, or persecution as in schizophrenia. The mood symptoms include depressed mood, manic symptoms, irritable and aggressive behavior, and hallucinatory experiences. First rank symptoms of schizophrenia, such as auditory hallucinations or a belief that thought is being inserted into their mind and negative symptoms such as amotivation, not socializing are not very common. An important characteristic feature is that there is a common lucid interval (coherent periods) of 2.5-48 hours following the return to baseline after the last seizure and after that the onset of psychosis.

The risk factors are age above 30 years, localization-related epilepsy, bilateral seizure, or interictal foci, clustering of seizures, secondary generalization, and perhaps, a family history of mood disorders but not psychosis.

Chronic Interictal Psychosis

Chronic interictal psychosis (CIP) is present in more than 5% of patients with a history of uncontrolled seizures; they can develop an insidious onset of paranoid delusions and hallucinations called CIP.[6]

Chronic interictal psychosis is more like schizophrenia than PIP. It is characterized by less intense mood components and more of persecutory auditory hallucinations. Eventhough positive symptoms (delusions, hallucinations, and referentiality) are common, there is a higher incidence of negative symptoms such as increasing isolation, decreasing socialization, overall downward cognitive, social, functional drift, and mood blunting, especially in patients with TLE (31%). First-rank symptoms involving disintegration of mental boundaries are usually absent in CIP and thought disorder is uncommon. Religiosity also occurs in them. Also, cognitive decline is correlated with the incidence of negative symptoms in TLE.

Forced Normalization or Alternative Psychosis

Landolt introduced the concept of forced normalization (FN) in two patients who developed personality and mood changes, but not psychosis, in association with normalization of their electroencephalograms (EEGs).[7] FN is emergence of psychiatric symptoms on electrical stabilization of the EEG. Alternative psychosis applies to the clinical phenomenon of a reciprocal relationship between abnormal mental states and seizures that did not rely on EEG findings. Paradoxical normalization describes epilepsy that is still active, but which remains subcortical.

Diagnostic criteria include: (1) epilepsy substantiated by history and EEG recordings, (2) new behavioral disturbances, (3) reduction by half in the number of EEG spikes, (4) a 1-week absence of seizures, (5) similar previous episodes, and (6) occurrence of such events on changes in antiepileptic pharmacotherapy.

Some of the explanations for FN include: (1) disinhibition of the limbic system after gaining seizure control and (2) limbic kindling. The kindling induced by electric or neurotransmitter processes is considered to result in these behavioral changes. Repeated limbic stimulation, mainly at the amygdala, olfactory bulb, and pyriform cortex appeared to create a behavioral action followed by motor responses. It is also hypothesized that chemical kindling causes behavioral issues, while electric kindling causes motor seizures.

De Novo Psychosis after Epilepsy Surgery

The prevalence rates range from <1% to 28.5%, with a mean of 7%. The most common psychiatric complication of temporal lobectomy is depression.

There are few reports of hypersexuality (excessive masturbation, social disinhibition), hyperphagia, and hyperthermia. Klüver–Bucy syndrome (KBS), which includes psychic blindness or visual agnosia, hypersexuality, emotional behavioral changes, such as placidity (decreased motor and verbal reaction against conditions that cause fear and anger), hyperorality (oral tendency, or compulsion to examine objects by mouth), and hypermetamorphosis (increased interest in every object that enters the visual field) is also associated with postepileptic surgery. Transient postoperative psychosis is typical and may be missed if not specifically assessed during the high-risk period of the first 6 months after surgery. The risk factors include a family history of psychosis, surgery after the age of 30 years, and preoperative psychosis.

MANAGEMENT

The mainstay of treatment is atypical antipsychotics because of their better side effect profile. Mood symptoms also can be managed with antidepressants, which improve the associated depression. Drug-to-drug interactions need to be monitored under such conditions.

PERSONALITY IN PERSONS WITH EPILEPSY

TEMPORAL LOBE EPILEPSY

Personality changes in TLE during the interictal periods have been described as early as the 19th century. They included hyposexuality (lack of sex drive or interest in engaging in sexual activity), hyper-religiosity (excessive interest in the cosmic and supernatural), hypergraphia (detailed accounts of daily events being recorded), and viscosity (interpersonal adhesiveness). Ongoing interictal abnormal electrical activity in the limbic system was found to be the reason for the behavioral changes.

There is an increased risk of violence and aggression in patients with epilepsy. Numerous studies have reported interictal aggression rates of 30% in TLE. Some of the risk factors for aggression in TLE included male gender, low IQ, lower socioeconomic status, and interruption of formal schooling. In fact, ictal and interictal aggression appear to be more common in children than in adults.

JUVENILE MYOCLONIC EPILEPSY

Janz[8] described personality changes with generalized epilepsies. The change noticed in juvenile myoclonic epilepsy (JME) includes irresponsibility, poor impulse control, neglect of self and duties, distractible, emotional instability, and inconsideration. They also have poor sleep habits, like late to bed and waking up late and sleep deprivation. These behaviors lead to poor compliance and make it difficult to manage epilepsy. Studies also report that patients with JME do less well on frontal lobe tasks than matched controls with TLE. Also, neuroimaging studies have shown subtle frontal lobe structural changes.

ABSENCE EPILEPSY

Previously considered as a benign form of epilepsy, absence epilepsy is associated with significant behavioral changes. A study by Wirrell et al.[9] reported that persons with absence seizures had significant difficulties in academics and also had behavioral problems compared to juvenile rheumatoid arthritis patients.

FRONTAL LOBE EPILEPSY

Frontal lobe epilepsy (FLE) is associated with alteration in personality, judgment, drive-related behavior, emotions, and executive functions. Anterior cingulate seizure foci are associated with antisocial behavior, recurrent intense sexual urges, sexually arousing fantasies, or behavior involving use of a nonhuman object, aggression, irritability, poor impulse control, interictal psychosis, and obsessive compulsive disorder (OCD). Orbitofrontal lesions can cause hyperphagia, failure to use autonomic cues to guide behavior, aberrant emotional responsiveness, increased aggression, dysfunctional social behavior, and behavioral disinhibition. Confabulation (memory disorders in which made-up stories fill in any gaps in memory) and attention-deficit hyperactivity disorder (ADHD) have been observed in the interictal period. Lopez-Rodriguez et al.[10] found cluster B (dramatic/emotional) or cluster C (anxious/fearful) personality disorders in FLE. However, it was not significantly different from TLE.

CONCLUSION

Persons' with epilepsy have associated psychiatric co-morbidities such as depression, anxiety disorders, psychosis and may exhibit personality changes. Psychiatric symptoms have a significant impact on their well-being and quality-of-life. Early recognition and management can lead to significant improvement in their quality-of-life. Psychotropics drugs should be used cautiously, as some of their adverse effects can interfere with the control of epilepsy and in a few cases may even lower seizure threshold.

REFERENCES

1. Elger CE, Johnston SA, Hoppe C. Diagnosing and treating depression in epilepsy. Seizure. 2017;44:184-93.

2. Fiest KM, Dykeman J, Patten SB, et al. Depression in epilepsy: a systematic review and meta-analysis. Neurology. 2013;80(6):590-9.
3. Sheline YI, Wang PW, Gado MH, et al. Hippocampal atrophy in recurrent major depression. Proc Natl Acad Sci USA. 1996;93(9):3908-13.
4. Gilliam FG, Barry JJ, Hermann BP, et al. Rapid detection of major depression in epilepsy: a multicentre study. Lancet Neurol. 2006;5(5):399-405.
5. Hoppe C, Elger CE. Depression in epilepsy: a critical review from a clinical perspective. Nat Rev Neurol. 2011;7(8):462-72.
6. Trimble MR. The Psychoses of Epilepsy. New York: Raven Press Publishers; 1991.
7. Landolt H. Serial EEG investigations during psychotic episodes in epileptic patients and during schizophrenic attacks. In: Lorentz de Haas AM (Ed). Lectures on Epilepsy. Amsterdam: Elsevier; 1958. pp. 91-133.
8. Janz D. The psychiatry of idiopathic generalized epilepsy. Neuropsychiatry Epilepsy. 2002;15:41-61.
9. Wirrell EC, Camfield CS, Camfield PR, et al. Long-term psychosocial outcome in typical absence epilepsy. Sometimes a wolf in sheeps' clothing. Arch Pediatr Adolesc Med. 1997;151(2):152-8.
10. Lopez-Rodriguez F, Altshuler L, Kay J, et al. Personality disorders among medically refractory epileptic patients. J Neuropsychiatry Clin Neurosci. 1999; 11(4):464-9.

9
Genetics of Epilepsy

Shishir Duble, Sanjib Sinha, Satishchandra P

INTRODUCTION

Over 50 million population worldwide are affected with epilepsy.[1] It is necessary that the recognition, approach to, and timely management of this condition shall remarkably improve the general well-being of the affected individuals in most of the cases. More than 50% of the population with epilepsy has a genetic basis.[2] However, unraveling the mysteries of genetics may be complex. In the last 2-3 decades, there has been a colossal change and advances in epilepsy genetics. From the time of discovering the first gene attributed to the causation of epilepsy—the *CHRNA4* gene—in 1995 to newer gene discoveries for epilepsy, made largely, due to advent of *newer* techniques including next generation sequencing (NGS) as well as collaborations in research with the Epilepsy Phenome/Genome Project (EPGP), Epi4K, and the EuroEPINOMICS-RES.[3] Over the last 2 decades, epilepsy genetics has evolved with the finding of de novo mutations, to one syndrome with multiple genes involved (genetic heterogeneity) and multiple phenotypes of one gene (pleitropy) with deciphering of new epilepsy syndromes. The most impressive findings have been made in relation to a greater integration of genetics into personalised treatment of individual patients.

GENETIC BASIS OF EPILEPSY

Genetic epilepsy denotes the form of epilepsy, which is due to a known or presumed genetic defect in which seizures are the important manifestation of the disease. In the recent International League Against Epilepsy (ILAE) 2017 classification of epilepsy, genetic syndromes have been incorporated in the etiology of epilepsy.[4]

Primarily, genetic diagnosis of epilepsy may be considered, when there is a history of epilepsy in the family. For example, history suggestive of autosomal dominant inheritance in case of benign familial neonatal convulsions. Secondly, studies on familial aggregation and twins have given humongous evidence of a genetic basis of epilepsy. Concordance rate for epilepsy is around 50-60% and 15% in monozygotic and dizygotic twins, respectively as revealed by twin studies. Concordance was found to be higher in generalized as compared to focal epilepsy. Seizure risk increases by eightfold and 2.5-fold in first-degree relatives with genetic generalized and focal epilepsies, respectively.[5] Most had only one other affected individual. There is a 3.3-fold increase in risk of having epilepsy in first-degree relatives of people living with epilepsy (4.7%) as compared to general population.[5]

Third, molecular genetics is assisting in identification of the underlying mutation, frequently de novo, in around 30-50% of infants with developmental/epileptic encephalopathies. For example, in Dravet syndrome, more than 80% have pathogenic variant in *SCN1A* gene. These mutations may lead to spectrum of epilepsies which range from febrile seizure, genetic epilepsy with febrile seizures plus (GEFS+), and Dravet syndrome with possible implications for treatment.[6]

Does Genetic Always Mean Inherited?

There is a wrong notion among patients and their relatives that genetic diseases are usually inherited. The word "genetic" does not always mean inherited. Clinical exome sequencing, targeted epilepsy gene, and Sanger sequencing have led to identification of increasing number of de novo mutations (sporadic or novel) both in mild and severe epilepsies. This means that the patient has a genetic alteration for the first time and, therefore is least likely to have inherited the mutation. At the same time, this patient now has a heritable mutation and is capable of transmission to offspring depending on type of de novo mutation.[7] For example, there is a 50% risk of having the mutation in those with dominant mutation. Nevertheless, the type of epilepsy and its expression might depend on the penetrance and variable expressivity of the mutation.[7] Furthermore, a patient may be mosaic for the mutation. In reference to mosaicism, person has two unique population of cells, with one population having the pathogenic variant mutation and the other having the wild type (normal) allele. Lower mosaicism rates result in milder form of epilepsy as shown in SCN1A studies.[6]

Disorder may be autosomal dominant in some and sporadic in others as a result of locus heterogeneity (identical disorder occurring in different families due to mutations in different genes, and each gene independently acting for the genesis of disease). Also, same gene mutation may result in different expressions among individuals (variable expressivity). *SCN1A* mutation has been detected in typical febrile seizures, GEFS+, Dravet syndrome, idiopathic generalized epilepsy (IGE), temporal lobe epilepsy, and Doose syndrome.[6] This variable expressivity in all probabilty results from the interaction of other genes or environmental factors.

MENDELIAN AND NONMENDELIAN INHERITANCE

Genetic causes of epilepsy may be divided into Mendelian (monogenic) inheritance and complex (polygenic) inheritance. Mendelian inheritance accounts for 1-2% of total genetic-related epilepsies.[7] Examples of dominant disorders are benign familial neonatal epilepsy (BFNE) and autosomal dominant nocturnal frontal lobe epilepsy (ADNFLE), where 50% of first-degree relatives will have the mutated gene. Recessive epilepsies are usually quite severe disorders (e.g. Lafora disease, Unverricht-Lundborg disease) with risk to siblings being 25% and should be considered in consanguineous parentage; X-linked disorders need a proper pedigree and are difficult to point out. Table 1 shows list of genetic epilepsies based on mode of inheritance.

EPILEPSY WITH COMPLEX INHERITANCE OR NONMENDELIAN

Genetic risk has additive effect on environmental factors. Multiple genes contribute to these traits, hence "polygenic", and also multiple environmental factors contribute, hence are also called "multifactorial". Multiple genes, which contribute to the disease, have a mild additive effect on the disease. None of the genes will have a single major effect on disease risk.[7] There may not be family history in any of these patients, and patient may appear surprised on revealing the cause as genetic. Individuals with polygenic etiologies, may have spontaneous seizures, while others have seizures only with additional environmental triggers, such as increased temperature, viral illness, alcohol ingestion, or sleep deprivation.

MITOCHONDRIAL INHERITANCE

Seizures are present in approximately 35-60% of mitochondrial (mt) dysfunction.[8] Around 30% of the refractory epilepsy are noted in confirmed mitochondrial dysfunction. Though seizures may be the presenting complaints in mitochondrial disease, it is usually suspected in the presence of systemic involvement such as sensorineural hearing loss (SNHL), diabetes mellitus, pigmentary retinopathy, liver disease, cardiomyopathy or cardiac conduction defects, and renal tubulopathy. Mutations in mtDNA and nuclear genes result in epilepsy. Seizures of explosive onset, epilepsia partialis continua and new-onset status epilepticus refractory to treatment, and occipital epileptiform discharges with photoparoxysmal responses are suspicious of mitochondrial etiology. Mitochondrial disease may also manifest as an early-onset epileptic encephalopathy, severe myoclonic disease, infantile spasms, and Lennox-Gastaut syndromes.[8] Children with

Table 1: Genetic epilepsy syndromes based on mode of inheritance.		
Mode of inheritance	Age of onset	Genes
Autosomal dominant:		
• BFNE	Birth to 1 month	KCNQ2, KCNQ3, and SCN2A
• BFIS	3–12 months	PRRT2, SCN2A, SCN8A, and CHRNA2
• ADFLE	First 2 decades	CHRNA4, CHRNA2, and CHRNB2
• ADPEAF/ADLTE	4–50 years	LGI1
• Familial focal epilepsy with variable foci (FFEVF)	3 months–24 years (variable)	DEPDC5
• GEFS+	6 months–6 years	SCN1A, SCN1B, and GABRG2
• Tuberous sclerosis	6 months–6 years	TSC1 and TSC2
• ADJME	5–16 years	GABRA1, EFHC1
Autosomal recessive:		
• ULD	6–15 years	Cystatin B mutation
• Lafora disease	Usually 8–18 years	NHLRC1, EPM2A mutation
• Neuronal ceroid lipofuscinosis	Before 6 years	CLN (1–8) mutations
X-linked disorders:		
• X-linked recessive—Boys only	As early as 1 month	ARX-related epilepsies
• X-linked dominant—Girls affected, boys severely affected:		
– Double cortex syndrome	Variable	DCX
– Periventricular nodular heterotopia	• Males—could be perinatally lethal	FLNA
	• Females—within the 1st year of life	
	3–19 years	PCDH19
PCDH19-related disorders:		
• Girls only (X-linked mental retardation limited to females)		
Mitochondrial inheritance:		
• MERRF	7–21 years	m.8344A>G, m.8356T>C, m.8363G>A, and m.8361G>A
• MELAS	14–39 years	m.3243A>G, m.13513G>A, m.3271T>C, and m.3252A>G
• Alpers syndrome	Birth to 7 years	POLG
• MEMSA	Variable	POLG

(ADFLE: autosomal dominant frontal lobe epilepsy; ADJME: autosomal dominant juvenile myoclonic epilepsy; ADLTE: autosomal dominant lateral temporal lobe epilepsy; ADPEAF: autosomal dominant partial epilepsy with auditory features; BFIS: benign familial infantile seizure; BFNE: benign familial neonatal epilepsy; GEFS+: genetic epilepsy with febrile seizures plus; MELAS: mitochondrial encephalopathy, lactic acidosis, and stroke-like episodes; MEMSA: myoclonic epilepsy myopathy sensory ataxia; MERRF: myclonic epilepsy with ragged-red fibers; PCDH19: protocadherin 19; ULD: Unverricht-Lundborg disease) epilepsy had a significantly higher incidence of complex I, III, and IV defects than children without epilepsy. *POLG* mutations range from Alpers syndrome to juvenile and adult-onset myoclonic epilepsy. Defective *POLG* mutations affects particularly complex I activity.

EPIGENETICS

Epigenetics refers to any structural change to the chromatin template that leads to functional changes in terms of gene expression, includes deoxyribonucleic acid (DNA) methylation, histone modifications, chromatin remodeling, and noncoding ribonucleic acids (RNAs). They contribute to the epileptogenic memory in difficult-to-treat epilepsies. Also, it may be used as biomarkers for progression of disease and as predictors for pharmacoresponsiveness.[9]

Are Genetic Epilepsies Always Nonlesional?

There is a common misunderstanding among physicians and neurologists that genetic epilepsy equals to a normal neuroimaging. It is not the case. These patients with structural pathology in MRI brain or nonspecific pathology are never evaluated for a genetic cause. Epilepsies, which are due to an obvious brain abnormality, are either due to genetic variation or external factors acting prenatally or after birth. Focal cortical dysplasia or a hypoxic ischemic damage is considered as the etiology of seizures. Given an example, in the case of a patient with severe intellectual disability and epilepsy with a relatively small lesion on MRI, do we still consider responsible for the symptoms? The answer to this query would be difficult, because in these group of patients, it will be difficult to classify them into either nongenetic, idiopathic/symptomatic, or genetic. More so, these group of patients may not be evaluated for any genetic studies.[10] In practice, lesional epilepsy is more common as compared to nonlesional ones. Some of the genetically determined lesional epilepsies include tuberous sclerosis (*TSC1* and *TSC2* mutations), double cortex syndrome (*DCX* mutation), and periventricular nodular heterotopia (*FLNA* mutation).

Why to Search for a Genetic Cause?

"Doctor, if you cannot cure my child's ailment completely, then how will doing genetic tests help?"—this is frequently asked by many family members. Genetic epilepsy was considered noncurable, however, views have changed. Though we have not yet reached a stage where finding a causative gene mutation has resulted in direct therapeutic consequences, genetic testing has somehow improved the management from treating epileptic encephalopathy due to glucose transporter type 1 (*GLUT1*) deficiency with

Table 2: Currently available/hypothesized precision medicine therapies.[11]

Conditions	Gene mutations	Treatment	Status of precision
Glucose transporter deficiency	SLC2A1	Ketogenic diet	Established
Pyridoxine-dependent epilepsy	ALDH7A1	Pyridoxine	Established
Migrating partial seizures of infancy	KCNT1	Quinidine or sodium channel blocker (carbamazepine)	Potential
Epileptic encephalopathy	KCNQ2	Ezogabine, sodium channel blockers	Established
Early-onset epileptic encephalopathy	GRIN2A	Memantine	Hypothetical
Tuberous sclerosis	mTOR	Everolimus	Established
Dravet syndrome	SCN1A	Avoid sodium channel blockers, stiripentol, and fenfluramine	Established
Mitochondrial epilepsy	POLG mutation	Avoid valproate	Established
GATOR1 complex	DEPDC5, NPRL2, and NPRL3	Mammalian target of rapamycin (mTOR) inhibitors	Hypothetical
Epileptic encephalopathy	KCNA2 mutation	4-aminopyridine	Hypothetical
Epileptic encephalopathy	SCN2A	Sodium channel blockers	Potential
Epileptic encephalopathy	SCN8A	Sodium channel blockers	Potential

ketogenic diet and withholding sodium channel blocker (e.g. lamotrigine) in Dravet syndrome. Table 2[11] showing overview of currently available/hypothesized precision medicine therapies in genetic epilepsies.

In a patient with untreatable epilepsy, also the parents/caretakers will be able to know the final diagnosis as genetic and also not relate epilepsy to minor head injury/infections/vaccination. Finding etiology of epilepsy reduces the burden of the relatives and decreases unwanted tests, which will be carried out in search of diagnosis. A genetic diagnosis will help in prognostication of disease and also know the natural history of disease (e.g. *PCDH19*-related epilepsy and Dravet syndrome). Lastly, genetic diagnosis helps in precise counseling with respect to the risk status of family members.[12]

The individual risk to a family member can be ascertained as in cases of familial epilepsy with a known single mutation. De novo mutations provide a challenge, since the risk to a further child is low, but not zero because of the possibility of parental mosaicism, which cannot easily be investigated. Counseling is also challenging when risk alleles (as opposed to genes determining Mendelian epilepsies) are detected. Currently, this is a rare practical problem as few risk alleles are known.

When to Suspect Clinically of Genetic Cause of Epilepsy?

Assessment of phenotype as well as meticulous patient and family history guide us in genetic testing. Certain points to be considered while considering a genetic cause:
- *Chromosomal*:
  - Three or more miscarriages in mother
  - Older age of mother (risk of aneuploidy)
  - Child's condition span multiple organ systems with presence of dysmorphic features
- *Autosomal dominant*:
  - Elderly paternal age
- *Autosomal recessive*:
  - Consanguineous parentage
  - Same geographic isolate
- *Disorders of genomic imprinting*:
  - Conceived through intracytoplasmic sperm injection (ICSI) or *in vitro* fertilization
- *Inborn error of metabolism*:
  - Increased urinary ketones
  - Hypoglycemia, anion gap acidosis, and hyperammonemia
  - Medically refractory epilepsy/neonatal seizures without definitive cause
  - Developmental regression
- *Mitochondrial*:
  - Developmental regression
  - Multisystem system/multiorgan involvement, including brain, heart, nerve/muscle, eyes, hearing, kidney, liver, etc.
  - Medically refractory epilepsy

Also, a diagnostic approach for evaluation of genetic epilepsy is shown in Flowchart 1.

PHARMACOGENETICS OF EPILEPSY

The difficulties experienced in the treatment of epilepsy, including refractoriness, adverse events, and unpredictability are partly genetically mediated. Functional polymorphisms in genes encoding drug target

Flowchart 1: Diagnostic testing in case of suspected genetic epilepsy.

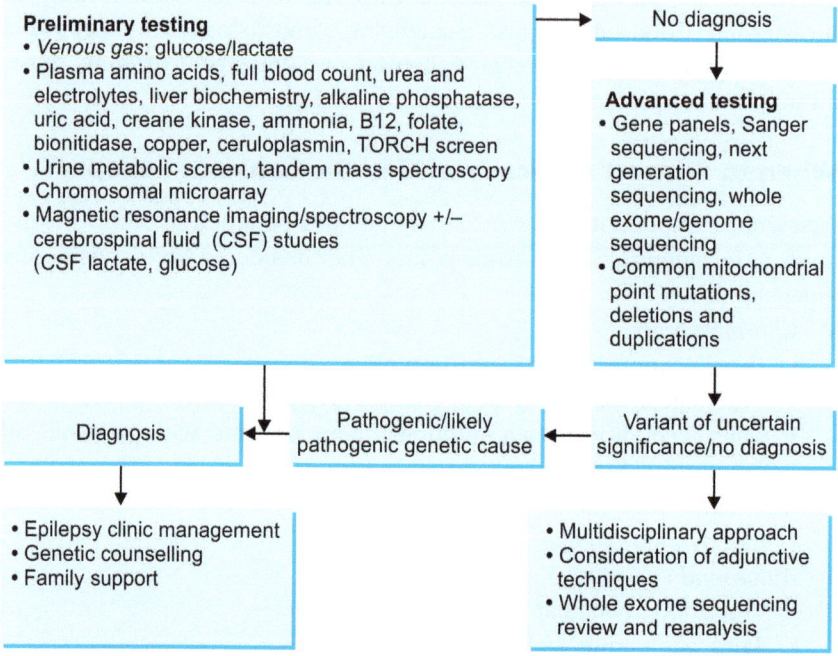

(*SCN1A*), drug transport (*ABCB1*), drug metabolizing (*CYP2C9*, *CYP2C19*), and human leukocyte antigen (HLA) proteins affect both pharmacokinetic and pharmacodynamics properties of antiseizure medications. This approach helps in guiding antiepileptic drug (AED) therapy and predicting early identification of potential side effects with treatment responsiveness before initiation, based on the patient's genotype. AED treatment commonly known to result in adverse drug reactions (ADRs). These events were not related to the number of AEDs but is due to type of AED used and individual susceptibility.

HLA-B*1502 is found to be a biomarker for Stevens–Johnson syndrome (SJS). In a study by Aggarwal et al., HLA-B*1502 is a risk factor for carbamazepine-induced SJS among patients from North India.[13] Proper screening for HLA-B*1502 prior to carbamazepine therapy in patients from Southeast Asia seems to be widely accepted and practiced to prevent SJS. There are various other AED biomarkers under research before validating clinical usage (multidrug resistance gene 1/*MDR1*/*ABCB1*/*PGY1*, *CYP2C9*, *CYP2C19*, *SCN1A*, *SCN2A*, *SCN3A*, and HLA-A*3101).

CHALLENGES IN GENETIC TESTING

Currently, the challenge in novel genetic testing in practice involves interpretation of the humongous amount of variants detected and data generated thereby. This results in difficulties to differentiate benign polymorphisms from risk factors or pathogenic mutations. Understanding the results requires proper phenotype and always needs to be performed in the context of the electroclinical syndrome and necessarily requires parenteral testing. Also, it has to be noted that detection of mutation also depends on type of mutation detection testing used; for example, Sanger sequencing versus NGS. In certain cases, it may be complementary to each other.

Negative testing for a particular gene does not rule out clinical diagnosis as other genes may be involved. Always a pretesting genetic counseling has to be done, which explained about the potential benefit and harms, possible limitations of test.

CONCLUSION

Epilepsy has a predominant genetic contribution; however, disentangling the genetic contribution can be tedious. There is lack of understanding of basic molecular pathophysiological processes underlying epileptogenesis. Genetic testing needs to be integrated into clinical decision making and is accompanied by several challenges including clinician education, interpretation of results, and counseling of parents and their families.

There is a recent shift in the genetic evaluation from research to clinical realm. Though, diagnostic tools including chromosomal microarray (CMA), gene panel testing, and whole exome sequencing (WES) have become readily available, they are inaccessible to some patients due to financial constraints and lack of awareness among physicians.

However, there is a ray of hope in everything we do as humans. The cost of genetic testing has dropped down remarkably to a price affordable to the present standard of living and there are many project-based centers opting to workup the patient on academic basis, free of cost. Genetic testing should become a part of our clinical practice as clinicians. On the outset, as precision therapies are emerging to a large extent genetic literacy, indeed is mandatory not only for the epileptologist but for the physicians.

REFERENCES

1. World Health Organization (WHO) (2010). Epilepsy in the WHO Eastern Mediterranean Region: Bridging the gap. [online] Available from https://apps.who.int/iris/bitstream/handle/10665/119905/dsa1039.pdf?sequence=1&isAllowed=y. [Last accessed from April, 2019].
2. Pal DK, Pong AW, Chung AW. Genetic evaluation and counseling for epilepsy. Nat Rev Neurol. 2010;6(8):445-53.
3. EuroEPINOMICS-RES Consortium, Epilepsy Phenome/Genome Project, Epi4K Consortium. De novo mutations in synaptic transmission genes including DNM1 cause epileptic encephalopathies. Am J Hum Genet. 2014;95(4):360-70.

4. Fisher RS, Cross JH, D'Souza C, et al. Instruction manual for the ILAE 2017 operational classification of seizure types. Epilepsia. 2017;58(4):531-42.
5. Peljto AL, Barker-Cummings C, Vasoli VM, et al. Familial risk of epilepsy: a population-based study. Brain. 2014;137(Pt 3):795-805.
6. Depienne C, Trouillard O, Gourfinkel-An I, et al. Mechanisms for variable expressivity of inherited SCN1A mutations causing Dravet syndrome. J Med Genet. 2010;47(6):404-10.
7. Berkovic SF. Genetics of epilepsy in clinical practice. Epilepsy Curr. 2015;15(4):192-6.
8. Canafoglia L, Franceschetti S, Antozzi C, et al. Epileptic phenotypes associated with mitochondrial disorders. Neurology. 2001;56(10):1340-6.
9. Kobow K, Blümcke I. Epigenetics in epilepsy. Neurosci Lett. 2018;667:40-6.
10. Kurian M, Korff CM, Ranza E, et al. Focal cortical malformations in children with early infantile epilepsy and PCDH19 mutations: case report. Dev Med Child Neurol. 2018;60(1):100-5.
11. Reif PS, Tsai MH, Helbig I, et al. Precision medicine in genetic epilepsies: break of dawn? Expert Rev Neurother. 2017;17(4):381-92.
12. Poduri A, Sheidley BR, Shostak S, et al. Genetic testing in the epilepsies-developments and dilemmas. Nat Rev Neurol. 2014;10(5):293-9.
13. Aggarwal R, Sharma M, Modi M, et al. HLA-B*1502 is associated with carbamazepine induced Stevens-Johnson syndrome in North Indian population. Hum Immunol. 2014;75(11):1120-2.

10
Investigations in Epilepsy

Viswanathan LG, Satishchandra P, Sanjib Sinha

INTRODUCTION

Epilepsy is one of the most commonly encountered neurological diseases in clinical practice for both physicians and neurologists. It is a condition wherein there is an enduring predisposition to suffer from recurrent seizures. Epilepsy is diagnosed when a person has two or more unprovoked/reflex seizures 24 hours apart or has had one seizure and has an underlying condition wherein the risk of recurrence is more than 60%.[1] The most valuable tool to diagnose a patient with epilepsy is a good clinical history from both the patient and witness. Extensive evaluation based on a poor history is ineffective and can be hazardous for both patient and treating physician. Diagnosing a patient with epilepsy has psychosocial/medical and legal implications. An array of investigations is available (Table 1), each having its unique indications and limitations. Knowledge regarding the same is essential prior to ordering these tests.

ELECTROENCEPHALOGRAPHY

Electroencephalography (EEG) is an essential tool in the evaluation and management of persons with epilepsy (PWE). EEG is a safe, noninvasive, and inexpensive test, which records the electrical activity that is generated in the brain over a period of time. Sensors, also called electrodes, are

Table 1: Investigations for a patient with epilepsy.	
Electrophysiology	EEG, video-EEG, magnetoencephalography
Imaging	MRI, PET, SPECT
Genetics	Karyotyping, chromosomal microarray, and next-generation sequencing
Other tests	• Biochemical tests • Electrophysiology • Neuropsychological assessment • Skin/muscle biopsy, etc.

(EEG: electroencephalography; MRI: magnetic resonance imaging; PET: positron emission tomography; SPECT: single-photon emission computed tomography)

applied over the scalp in a standardized pattern—called 10-20 system. The electrodes on the right side are numbered with even numbers and left-sided electrodes—odd (Fig. 1A). The electrical activity generated in the brain is in the range of microvolts (vis-à-vis millivolts in EKG). Thus, the recording is contaminated with noise and electrical activity generated elsewhere in the body and the environment (called artefacts). Numerous filters and amplifiers are used to modify these signals. In the modern era, EEG is displayed on computer monitors—called digital EEGs. Knowledge about filter settings and technical aspects are crucial to understand and report EEGs, which is out of the scope of this chapter. EEG is generally recorded for about half an hour and should ideally include eye opening and closure, hyperventilation, and photic stimulation. Events that occur during the recording should be marked by the technician for easier interpretation.

An EEG is only performed as a supportive investigative procedure, when epilepsy has been diagnosed/suspected based on clinical history. It cannot and should not be used as a standalone investigation to diagnose epilepsy or exclude its presence. EEG has a very wide sensitivity and specificity for diagnosing epilepsy. Ideally, the yield of EEG increases when it is performed soon after the last seizure (within 24-48 hours) or when it is performed in a sleep-deprived state.[2]

Interpretation of EEG requires adequate training and skill. Many physiological waveforms and artefacts may falsely be interpreted as abnormal by inexperienced physicians. There are a few prerequisites to be known prior to reading an EEG. These are the age of the individual, the state of consciousness, whether sleep is natural or sedated and if the patient was on any drugs at the time of recording the EEG. In this way, EEG supports the operational classification of the type of seizures associated with various types of epilepsy.

In population studies, only 32-59% of EEGs are abnormal after the first episode of seizure.[3] EEGs are more likely to be abnormal in patients who have had generalized seizures as compared to patients who have had focal seizures. The risk of recurrence of seizures, if the EEG shows abnormal interictal epileptiform discharges (IEDs) after the first episode, is about 60%[4] and, hence, requires treatment with antiepileptic drug (AED). The increase in relative risk of developing a second seizure is almost two times as compared to patients who did not exhibit EEG abnormalities after the first episode. Normal recordings are seen in nearly 30% of cases, and 10% of PWE have persistently normal EEG recordings.[5] The frequency of IEDs does not predict seizure response or therapeutic response. Normal individuals may show IEDs in EEG recordings (0.2-0.5% in adults and up to 3.5% in children).[6] However, the type of epileptiform discharge does have a bearing on the chances of seizures recurrence, e.g. generalized discharges and polyspikes

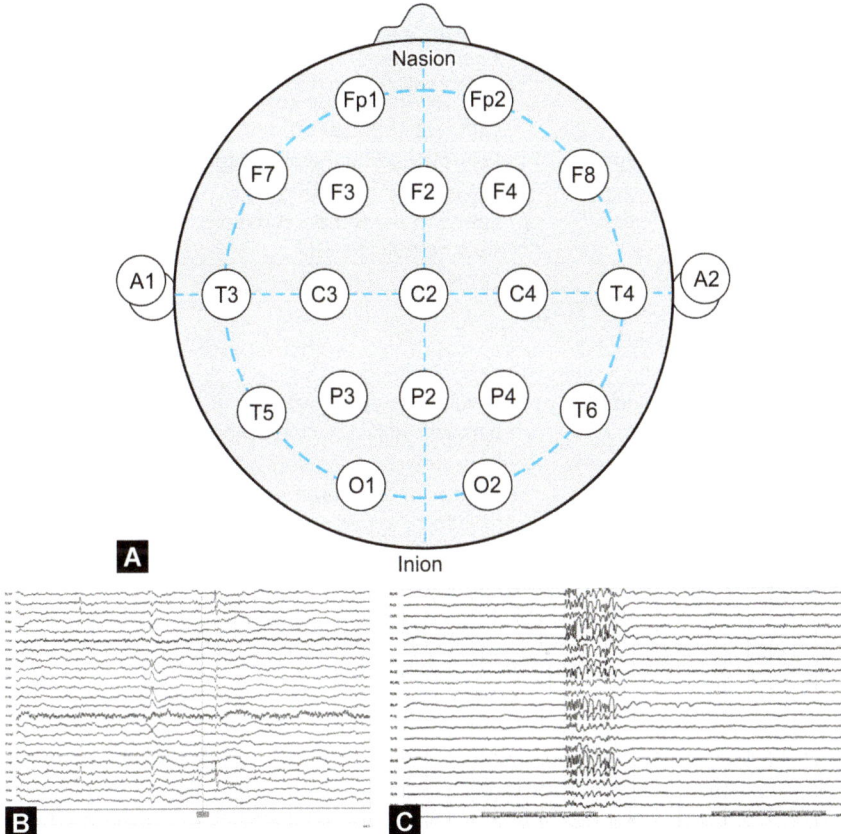

Figs. 1A to C: (A) The international 10–20 montage system. (B) A 26-year-old male presented with complex partial seizures. Average reference montage shows spikes are seen in the right anterior temporal leads (T2, T4, F10, and F8). On evaluation, patient had right hippocampal sclerosis. (C) A 26-year-old lady presented with myoclonic jerks in the morning. Bipolar longitudinal montage shows generalized polyspike, spike, and wave discharge of about 4 Hz frequency during photic stimulation (photoparoxysmal response). Patient had juvenile myoclonic epilepsy.

are more likely to be epileptogenic. PWE who have generalized seizures may exhibit focal IEDs in EEG [as much as 30% in juvenile myoclonic epilepsy (JME)], especially during sleep. Awareness of this fact is crucial to avoid misdiagnosing the type of epilepsy by means of EEG.

Predicting a successful response to an AED is based on electroclinical features (Figs. 1B and C; and Table 2). The usefulness of EEG in predicting seizure recurrence before starting an AED taper in seizure-free patients is controversial. In patients who have been seizure free on AEDs for more than 2–5 years, tapering and possible cessation of AEDs may avoid adverse

Table 2: Electroencephalography (EEG) abnormalities in a few epileptic syndromes.	
Type of epilepsy	Characteristic EEG
Absence epilepsy	3 Hz generalized spike wave discharge, induced with hyperventilation
Juvenile myoclonic epilepsy	Polyspike and generalized spike wave discharges (>4 Hz) (see Fig. 1C)
Temporal lobe epilepsy	Spikes in the temporal region, intermittent focal slowing (see Fig. 1B)
Childhood epilepsy with centrotemporal spikes (CECTs, previously known as benign rolandic epilepsy)	Centrotemporal spikes
Lennox-Gastaut syndrome	Slow spike wave discharge (<2.5 Hz), generalized paroxysmal fast activity (seen in sleep)
West syndrome	Hypsarrhythmia (chaotic, disorganized, and high-amplitude asynchronous activity in the EEG with multifocal spikes and sharp waves)

effects from long-term use. With respect to individuals suffering from idiopathic generalized epilepsy (IGE), the presence of generalized spike and wave discharges (GSWD) in the EEG prior to AED taper suggests a greater likelihood of seizure relapse. This may warrant the need for continued treatment. Centrotemporal spikes (CTS) in the EEG of childhood epilepsy with CTS (CECTS) patients have good response to AEDs and commonly remit in adolescence. Patients with certain forms of epilepsy such as JME will require long-term AED treatment (possibly lifelong) and it may be wise to continue AEDs albeit at low dose, irrespective of EEG findings. Thus, rather than just using a normal EEG as an endpoint to taper AED, the successful withdrawal of AEDs depends on the timing of taper and the electroclinical syndrome.

OTHER ELECTROPHYSIOLOGICAL PROCEDURES

Apart from EEG, various other procedures are available to extend the evaluation of a PWE. VEEG or telemetry is the combined recording of EEG and video of the patient to characterize semiology and identify the region of onset of seizures. MEG or magnetoencephalography (Figs. 2A to D), stereo-EEG and invasive intracranial EEG are specialized procedures done for patients in centers that cater to patients with refractory epilepsy.

IMAGING MODALITIES

The diagnosis of epilepsy is clinical and though imaging is not crucial for its diagnosis, but is essential to identify the etiology and thus the prognosis. It is also very useful in patients who suffer from refractory seizures. Two

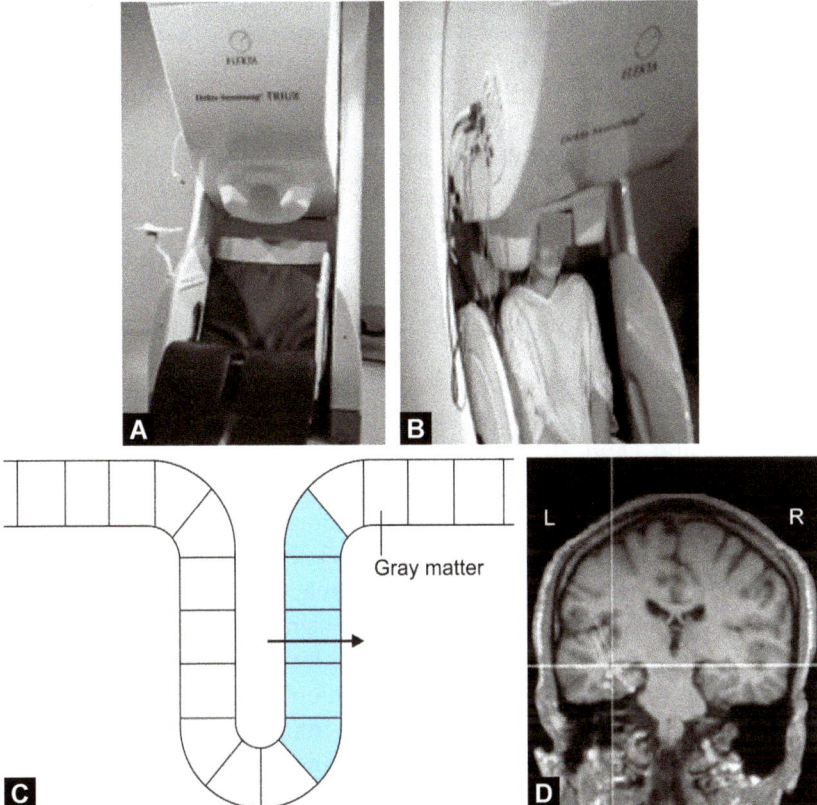

Figs. 2A to D: (A and B) The Elekta Neuromag® TRIUX magnetoencephalography (MEG) machine at NIMHANS and a patient undergoing MEG in a magnetically shielded room. (C) Tangential magnetic dipole in the gyrus, which is recorded by the MEG machine. (D) Equivalent current dipole (ECD) modeling of IED revealing dipole cluster: Dipole cluster in the left medial temporal lobe.

of the commonly available imaging modalities are computed tomography (CT) scan and magnetic resonance imaging (MRI). CT is widely available, cheaper than MRI, faster to acquire, and hence useful in acute setting. However, it exposes the individual to radiation and it is not a very sensitive tool to detect many anomalies in the brain. Nevertheless, it is still widely used in practice despite its limitations.

Magnetic Resonance Imaging

Magnetic resonance imaging is a useful imaging modality for evaluating PWE. MRI offers excellent spatial resolution (especially high-field strength machines—1.5T and 3T), good contrast between gray and white matter, and does not expose the patient to radiation. MRI uses a strong magnetic

Table 3: Epilepsy protocol magnetic resonance imaging (MRI).				
Sequence	Slice thickness	Plane	Axis	Findings
3D T1	1 mm	3D	Ac-pc	To look for gray-white junction
T2 STIR	<3 mm	Axial, coronal	Hc	Identifies areas of altered signal in lesions, hippocampal sclerosis
FLAIR	<3 mm	3D or axial, coronal	Hc	
SWI	<3 mm	Axial	Ac-pc	Calcifications, bleeds

(Hc: hippocampus; Ac-pc: anterior commissure-posterior commissure)

field and radiofrequency pulses to acquire images of the body, based on the concentration of protons in the imaged area. Commonly used sequences are T1, T2, and Fluid Attenuated Inversion Recovery (FLAIR) sequences; however, imaging protocols in epilepsy mandate the use of other special sequences such as a 3D T1 sequence, oblique coronal 3D FLAIR, and susceptibility weighted imaging. The slice thickness should be at least 3 mm, so that small lesions will not be missed (Table 3). MRI machines of low-field strength cannot maintain an adequate signal-to-noise ratio at such a small slice thickness and result in images with poor resolution, and hence must be considered obsolete in the evaluation of PWE. The objective of implementing various sequences is to obtain information regarding the site, extent, and nature of the lesion. Cursory examination of MRIs of patients suffering from epilepsy will not suffice. Careful scrutiny of the images will often reveal subtle abnormalities, often having significant implications with respect to patient care. Some of the common abnormalities that can be identified in PWE MRIs are listed in Table 4. Abnormal imaging after a first seizure (e.g. hippocampal sclerosis) is predictive of a high risk of recurrence of seizures and ascertains the diagnosis of epilepsy even after a single attack. Though the natural history of other lesions [e.g. focal cortical dysplasia (FCD)] (Figs. 3A and B) has not been systemically studied, experience suggests that the risk of recurrence is indeed high and patients would require further evaluation and AEDs after the first episode of seizure. Imaging in patients with idiopathic generalized epilepsy is usually normal.

All patients with epilepsy, especially those who are refractory to AEDs must undergo imaging with MRI, except those with very typical forms of IGE syndromes with characteristic EEG features and good response to AEDs.[7] The purpose of imaging is mainly to define the cause for epilepsy, more so when it is drug refractory as it may be surgically remediable. However, one must keep in mind that not all lesions found in the MRI are epileptogenic and focal epilepsies can be present in patients who have seemingly normal MRIs. This situation arises in individuals who have subtle malformations of cortical development such as FCD. MRI has a high sensitivity and specificity

Table 4: Magnetic resonance imaging (MRI) findings in certain epileptogenic lesions.	
Disease	Abnormality found
Mesial temporal lobe epilepsy	Reduction in hippocampal volumes, flattening of hippocampus, increased signal in T2 FLAIR sequence (Fig. 3A)
Focal cortical dysplasia (FCD)	Blurring of the gray-white junction, transmantle sign (Fig. 3B)
Calcification	Low signal on T2, iso in T1 and blooming in SWI
Ganglioglioma	Lesion with soap bubble appearance on T2

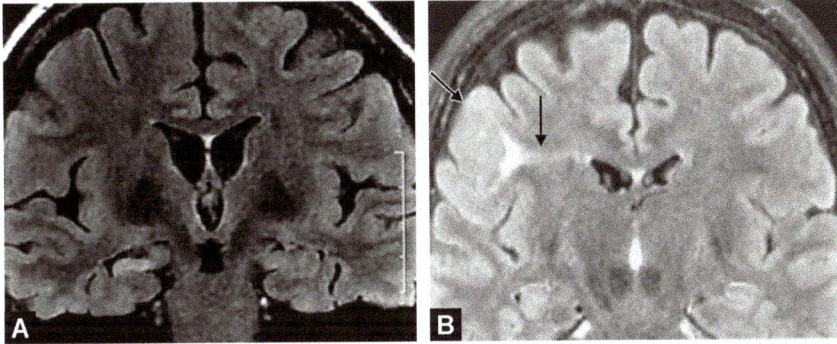

Figs. 3A and B: (A) FLAIR coronal sequence showing loss of volume and increased signal in the right hippocampus with slight dilation of the temporal horn—Right mesial temporal sclerosis (MTS). (B) FLAIR sequence showing hyperintensity in the right frontal region with poor gray-white differentiation and the "transmantle sign" suggestive of focal cortical dysplasia (FCD) type 2b.

for other lesions such as hippocampal sclerosis, vascular malformations, postischemic/traumatic lesions, inflammatory and infectious diseases, and tumors. MRI also allows quantitative analysis such as hippocampal volumetry, assessment of white matter tracts with DTI (diffusion tensor imaging), etc.

Other imaging modalities that are available are positron emission tomography (PET) (Figs. 4A and B) and single photon emission CT (SPECT) and functional imaging studies such as functional MRI (fMRI) (Figs. 5A and B).

OTHER INVESTIGATIONS FOR EPILEPSY

Drug levels of common AEDs such as phenytoin, phenobarbitone, carbamazepine, and valproate are widely available. These tests are useful when toxicity is suspected or when compliance is doubtful. It

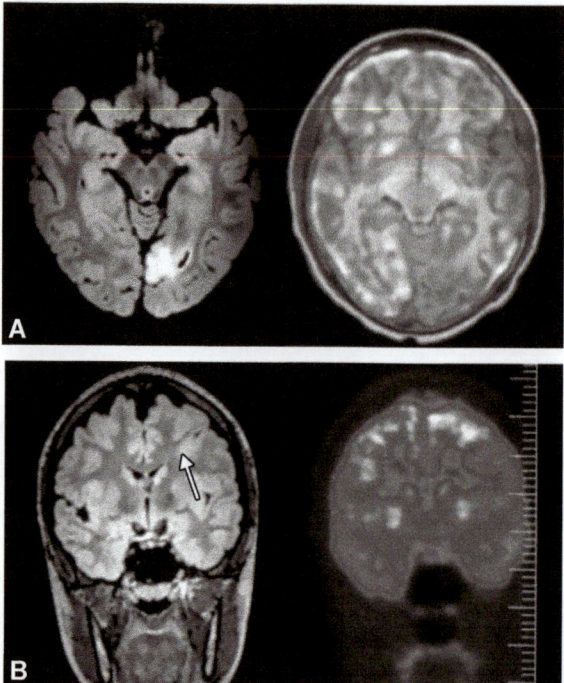

Figs. 4A and B: (A) T2 hyperintense lesion in the medial aspect of the left occipital lobe. Corresponding slice of the interictal positron emission tomography-magnetic resonance imaging (PET-MRI) shows severe hypometabolism in the same area. (B) Magnetic resonance imaging (MRI) shows a left frontal focal cortical dysplasia (FCD) and ictal PET-MR shows hypermetabolism of the left frontal region.

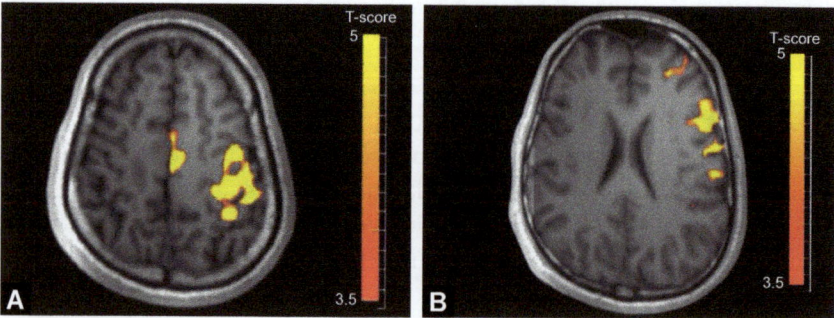

Figs. 5A and B: (A) Functional magnetic resonance imaging (fMRI) showing localization of the left motor cortex when patient is moving the fingers of the right hand (marked in yellow). (B) fMRI showing localization of the language areas, which are showing in yellow during a picture naming task.

may also be done when AEDs are coprescribed with drugs, which have significant interactions, which in turn will have a bearing on the steady state of drug levels in the blood. Many other modalities are available to evaluate epilepsy such as genetics, specialized biochemical investigations, and biopsy of skin and muscle (for conditions such as neuronal ceroid lipofuscinosis, mitochondrial syndromes, and Lafora body disease). Details for genetic evaluation of epilepsy have been given in Chapter 9 (Genetics of Epilepsy). Patients suffering from epilepsy commonly have cognitive and neuropsychological impairment, which can be assessed by formal neuropsychological testing. These deficits may be due to the underlying pathology, epilepsy syndrome, drug effects, and coexisting psychiatric illness or as a result of ongoing seizures.

CONCLUSION

Epilepsy is a chronic illness and is disabling in about 20–25% of patients appropriate evaluation and treatment at first contact with the patient can make a big difference in long-term care. A brief flowchart has been described in Flowcharts 1 and 2 regarding the approach to a patient with

Flowchart 1: Approach to evaluation of epilepsy with electroencephalography/magnetic resonance imaging (EEG/MRI).

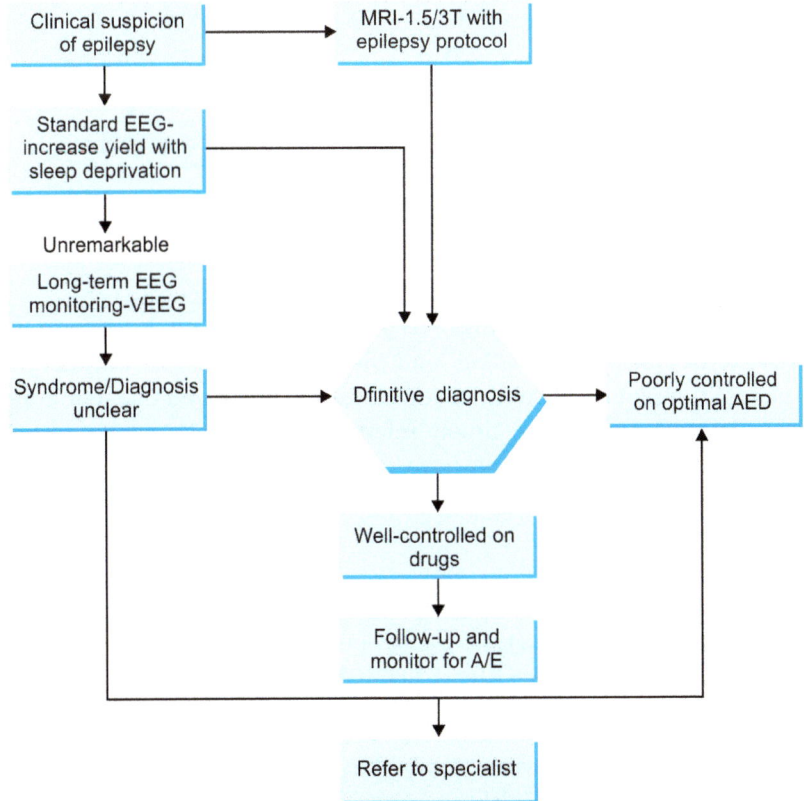

(AED: antiepileptic drug; VEEG: video electroencephalography)
Note: The diagnosis of epilepsy is clinical and not all patients would require MRI/EEG for a routine diagnosis. However, to classify patients into particular epilepsy syndromes, evaluation with EEG and imaging would be ideal.

Flowchart 2: Simplified approach to drug-resistant epilepsy.

```
                    Localization related epilepsy
                    ┌──────────────┴──────────────┐
            Lesion present                    MRI negative
              in MRI                              │
                │                              Video EEG
            Video EEG                              │
            concordant                             │
         ┌──────┴──────┐                           │
        Yes            No ──────────────→ MEG, PET/SPECT
         │                                         │
         │                                 Hypothesis reached?
         │                                 ┌───────┴───────┐
         │                                Yes              No
         │                                 │               │
         └─────────→ Plan for surgery ←────┘       Palliative interventions
```

(MEG: magnetoencephalography; PET: Positron emission tomography; SPECT: single-photon emission computed tomography)

epilepsy and refractory seizures, respectively. EEG and MRI form the backbone of epilepsy evaluation, and their judicious use is warranted to extract maximum benefit for the patient. It is reemphasized that a thorough history is most crucial and timely referral to a specialty center may be recommended in patients who have complicated epilepsy syndromes or when there is doubt in the diagnosis.

REFERENCES

1. Falco-Walter J, Scheffer I, Fisher R. The new definition and classification of seizures and epilepsy. Epilepsy Res. 2018;139:73-9.
2. King D, Spencer S, Bronen R, et al. EEG findings in patients with hippocampal atrophy. Neurology. 1998;50(5):1515-6.
3. Baldin E, Hauser W, Buchhalter J, et al. Yield of epileptiform electroencephalogram abnormalities in incident unprovoked seizures: a population-based study. Epilepsia. 2014;55(9):1389-98.
4. Berg A. Risk of recurrence after a first unprovoked seizure. Epilepsia. 2008;49 Suppl 1:13-8.

5. Shinnar S, Berg A, O'Dell C, et al. Predictors of multiple seizures in a cohort of children prospectively followed from the time of their first unprovoked seizure. Ann Neurol. 2000;48(2):140-7.
6. Pillai J, Sperling M. Interictal EEG and the diagnosis of epilepsy. Epilepsia. 2006;47(s1):14-22.
7. Berg A, Berkovic S, Brodie M, et al. Revised terminology and concepts for organization of seizures and epilepsies: Report of the ILAE Commission on Classification and Terminology, 2005-2009. Epilepsia. 2010;51(4):676-85.

11
Emergencies in Epilepsy: Diagnosis and Management

Shiva Kumar R

INTRODUCTION

Seizure is one of the most common neurological emergencies encountered in clinical practice. Seizures can happen at home, outside the home, or in hospital settings such as casualty, in-patient wards, and in the criticalcare units. Emergencies in epilepsy can be broadly categorized into cluster or acute repetitive seizures, convulsive status epilepticus (CSE), and nonconvulsive status epilepticus (NCSE). Timely diagnosis of these seizure emergencies is crucial for their successful management.

Types of emergencies in epilepsy are:
- Isolated seizures—first seizure or rare seizures
- Cluster seizures (acute repetitive seizures)
- Status epilepticus—convulsive or nonconvulsive.

CLUSTER SEIZURES (ACUTE REPETITIVE SEIZURES)

Acute repetitive seizures are the most common epilepsy emergencies seen in the casualty. Cluster seizures are defined as three or more seizures occurring within a 24-hour period with a return to baseline clinical condition between the attacks. Cluster seizures can last anywhere from a few minutes to up to a day. Cluster seizures increase the risk of occurrence of status epilepticus (SE) by nearly fourfold.

Risk of developing cluster seizures is high in people who have very high-seizure burden, severe forms of epilepsy, extratemporal epilepsies (mainly frontal), having longer duration of epilepsy, and with a history of recent worsening of pre-existing epilepsy.

Treatment of Acute Repetitive Seizures

- Using extra doses of usual antiepileptic medications
- Oral benzodiazepines (rectal or oral diazepam or oral clobazam)
- Nasal (midazolam available as 0.5 and 1.25 mg per nasal puff)

- Parenteral benzodiazepines (IM, buccal, or IV midazolam, IV lorazepam, and IV diazepam)
- Broad-spectrum parenteral anticonvulsants effective against multiple seizure types.

STATUS EPILEPTICUS

Status epilepticus (SE) is an underdiagnosed serious neurological emergency generally managed by neurophysicians, pediatricians, and general practitioners. SE is associated with significant morbidity and mortality and requires immediate treatment to stop the ongoing seizures to prevent neuronal cell injury or death.

Status epilepticus is classically defined as a single epileptic seizure, which lasts for more than 5 minutes or two or more seizures occurring within a 5-minute period without the person regaining consciousness in-between. For all practical purposes, SE should be considered in any one who is still convulsing in the emergency department.

Classification of Status Epilepticus

Like seizure classification, classification of SE is important in clinical practice for appropriate management of the condition because effective treatment depends on the type of SE. Depending on whether convulsive activity is present or not, SE is classified into CSE and NCSE. Convulsive SE is the most common and most serious form of epilepsy emergency associated with high mortality and morbidity.[1]

"Time is Brain" in Status Epilepticus

Like stroke, time is important ("Time is Brain") in the management of SE. Rapid and early treatment of SE helps in decreasing the morbidity and mortality. Hence, effective and timely treatment of SE has a decisive role for a good prognosis.

Epidemiology of Status Epilepticus

The occurrence of SE has bimodal distribution with most cases occurring in children less than 3 years of age and in the elderly (>60 years). Incidence of SE is variable and varies from region to region. In India and other developing countries, SE is more common due to higher incidence of central nervous system (CNS) and systemic infections, brain infestations such as cysticercosis, stroke (arterial and venous), and traumatic head injuries.[2] Treatment gap and poor compliance to anticonvulsant drugs in pre-existing epilepsy increase the risk of SE in developing countries (Box 1).

Box 1: Etiology of status epilepticus.

- *Known (i.e. symptomatic) causes:*
  - Acute (e.g. stroke, intoxication, malaria, encephalitis, etc.)
  - Remote (e.g. post-traumatic, postencephalitic, poststroke, etc.)
  - Progressive (e.g. brain tumor, Lafora's disease and other PMEs, dementias)
  - Status epilepticus defined electroclinical syndromes:
    - Myoclonic status in juvenile myoclonic epilepsy and Down syndrome
    - Absence status in juvenile absence epilepsy
    - Lennox-Gastuat syndrome, Panayiotopoulos syndrome, etc.
- *Unknown (i.e. cryptogenic) causes:*
  - De novo status epilepticus
  - NORSE—New onset refractory status epilepticus
  - FIRES—Febrile infection-related epilepsy syndrome

Source: Adapted from Trinka E, et al. Epilepsia 2015.

Prognostic Factors in Status Epilepticus

Outcome in the management of SE depends on the cause, duration, the treatment offered, and the age of the patient (children have better outcomes than adults).[3] Mortality from SE (which is defined as death within 30 days of SE) is highest in the elderly and is about 38%. Children have better prognosis compared to adults (3 vs 26%).[4]

Status epilepticus occurring after hypoxia ischemic injury and cerebral stroke has a very high mortality rate. SE occurring in the setting of alcohol withdrawal and low levels of antiepileptic drugs has good prognosis. Cognitive impairment and persistent seizures are the most common long-term complications seen after successful treatment of prolonged SE.

Management of Status Epilepticus

Medical Management of Status Epilepticus

Based on American Epilepsy Society, 2016 guidelines for management of SE, the treatment of SE is divided in to four phases:

Phase 1: 0-5 minute (stabilization phase):
- Stabilize airway, breathing, and circulation
- Time seizure from onset, monitor vital signs, and follow management protocol (Flowchart 1).

Phase 2: 5-20 minutes (initial therapy phase):
- First-line agents in SE treatment:
  - *Lorazepam:* 0.1 mg/kg/dose (maximum 4 mg/dose) IV over 2 minutes; if required dose can be repeated after 5 minutes
  - *Diazepam:* 0.15-0.2 mg/kg/dose (maximum 10 mg/dose) IV over 2 minutes; if required dose can be repeated after 5 minutes

Flowchart 1: Algorithm for management of convulsive and nonconvulsive status epilepticus.

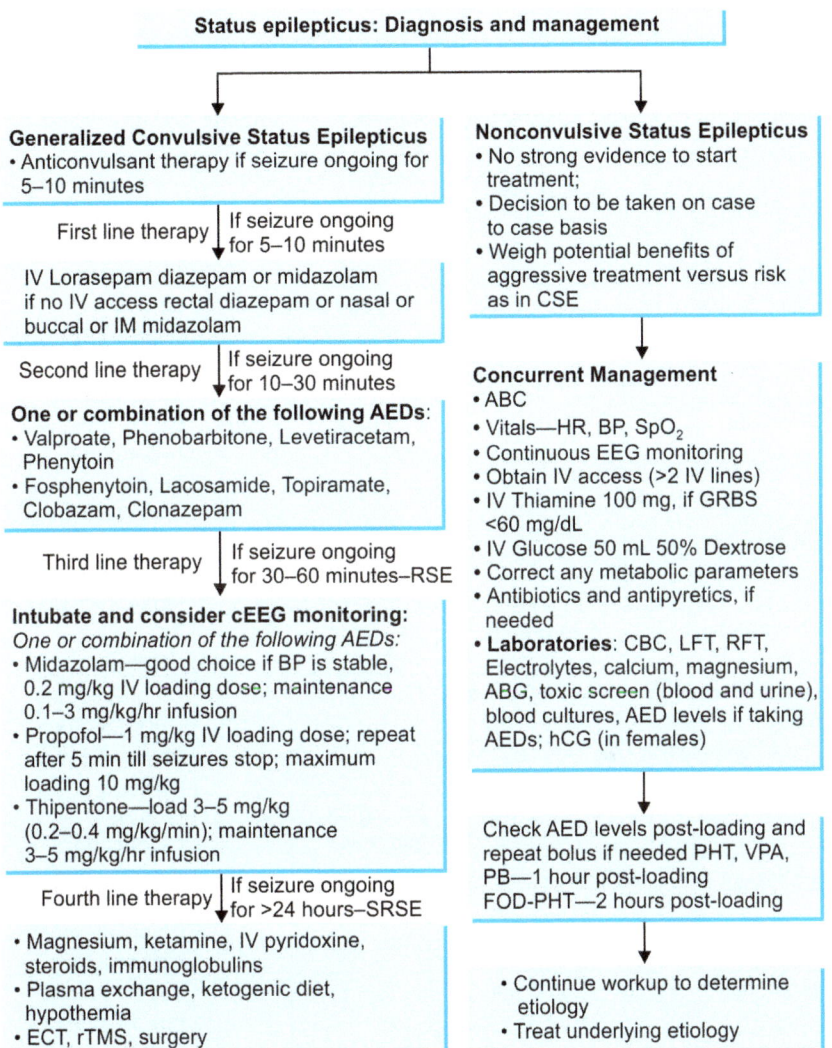

- *Midazolam*: 0.2 mg/kg/dose (maximum 10 mg/dose) IV over 2 minutes; if required dose can be repeated after 5 minutes till seizures subside or 10 mg IM single dose (if there is no IV access).
- *Monitor for respiratory rate (count respiratory rate for full 1 minute)*:
  - If the respiratory rate is less than 8 breaths/min, avoid benzodiazepines; start second-line therapy
  - If the respiratory rate is less than 4 breaths/min, prepare for mechanical ventilation.

Phase 3: 20-40 minutes (second-line therapy phase):
- See Table 1 and Flowchart 1 for AEDs in status epilepticus.

Table 1: First and second line antiepileptic drugs (AEDs) in status epilepticus (SE) and their pharmacokinetics.					
AEDs	Route	Loading dose	Maximum rate of infusion	Enzyme induction	Adverse effects
Phenytoin	IV	20 mg/kg	50 mg/min	Yes	Cardiac depression, hypotension
Fosphenytoin	IV or IM	20 mg/kg	150 mg/min	Yes	Cardiac depression, hypotension, paresthesias
Valproate	IV	40 mg/kg	6 mg/kg/min	Inhibition	Pancreatitis, hyperammonemia, encephalopathy, thrombocytopenia, deranged LFT, hepatotoxicity
Phenobarbitone	IV	20 mg/kg	50–75 mg/min	Yes	Respiratory depression
Levetiracetam	IV	20–60 mg/kg	100 mg/min	No	Fatigue, somnolence, transient thrombocytopenia
Lacosamide	IV	10–12 mg/kg	0.4 mg/kg/min	No	Cardiac conduction abnormalities, myoclonus, confusion, elevated liver enzymes
Topiramate	Oral	200–1,000 mg/kg	—	No	Hyperammonemia if combined with VPA; ataxia, confusion, cognitive impairment
Clobazam	Oral	10–40	—	No	Ataxia, vertigo, drowsiness
Clonazepam	Oral	1–4 mg	—	No	Respiratory and cardiac depression, increased secretions, paradoxical worsening of seizures

Phase 4: 40–60 minutes (third-line therapy phase) (refractory status epilepticus):
- If seizures continue, switch to other second-line drugs
- If refractory, consider anesthetic agents:
  - Midazolam, thiopental, pentobarbital, propofol, and ketamine
  - Inhalational anesthetic agents.

Super-Refractory Status Epilepticus

- If seizures persist beyond 24 hours of general anesthesia or recur upon reduction/withdrawal of general anesthesia.
- Any combination of the following, if situation demands:
  - IV Magnesium 4 mg bolus, then 2–6 g/hr
  - Ketamine load—1.5 mg/kg IV, repeat every 5 minutes till seizures stop (maximum loading 4.5 mg/kg; maintenance 1.2–7.5 mg/kg)
  - IV pyridoxine 200 mg/day
  - Immunomodulation—IV methylprednisolone 1 g × 3–5 days and or IV immunoglobulins 0.4 mg/kg/day × 5 days and or plasma exchange for 5–7 days
  - Ketogenic diet
  - Therapeutic hypothermia
  - Electroconvulsive therapy (ECT)
  - Transcranial magnetic stimulation (TMS)
  - Neurosurgical options, if feasible.

Note:
- If a patient is already on some anticonvulsant drug, same drug can be started initially in the treatment of SE.
- Antibiotics such as quinolones, third-generation cephalosporins, cefepime, and carbapenem can result in seizure exacerbation and can cause SE, especially in patients with impaired renal and hepatic functions.

Role of Electroencephalography

- In established convulsive SE, where the diagnosis is clinically apparent, EEG may not be required for establishing diagnosis
- Continuous electroencephalography (cEEG) is indicated in unexplained coma or altered sensorium after convulsive SE (at least 24 hour EEG to ensure that the recurrent and/or subtle SE are not missed)[5]
- For classification of SE
- Is suspected cases of pseudostatus epilepticus
- For diagnosis of NCSE (Figures 1A to D showing generalized NCSE and Figures 2A to D showing focal NCSE)
- Monitoring and maintaining burst suppression during the treatment of SE.

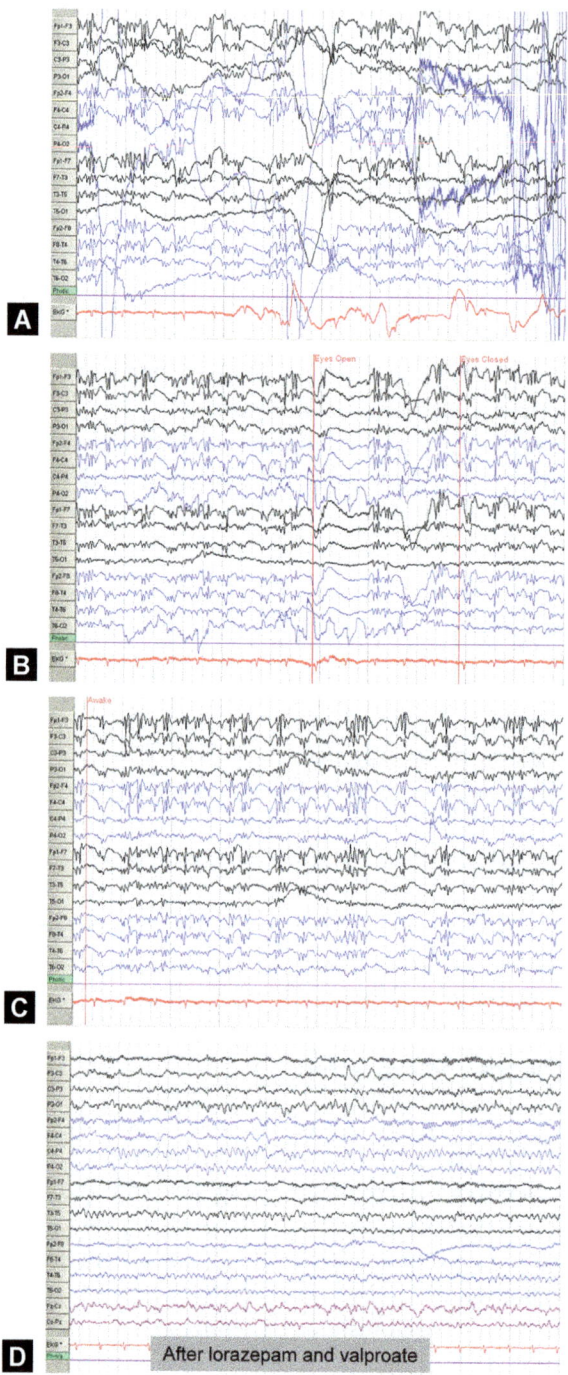

Figs. 1A to D: EEG showing myoclonic status in a patient when prescribed phenytoin in primary generalized epilepsy. (A to C) show spikes, polyspikes and wave discharges in a patient with multifocal jerks with preserved consciousness; (D) shows EEG with normal background activity after administration of lorazepam and valproate.

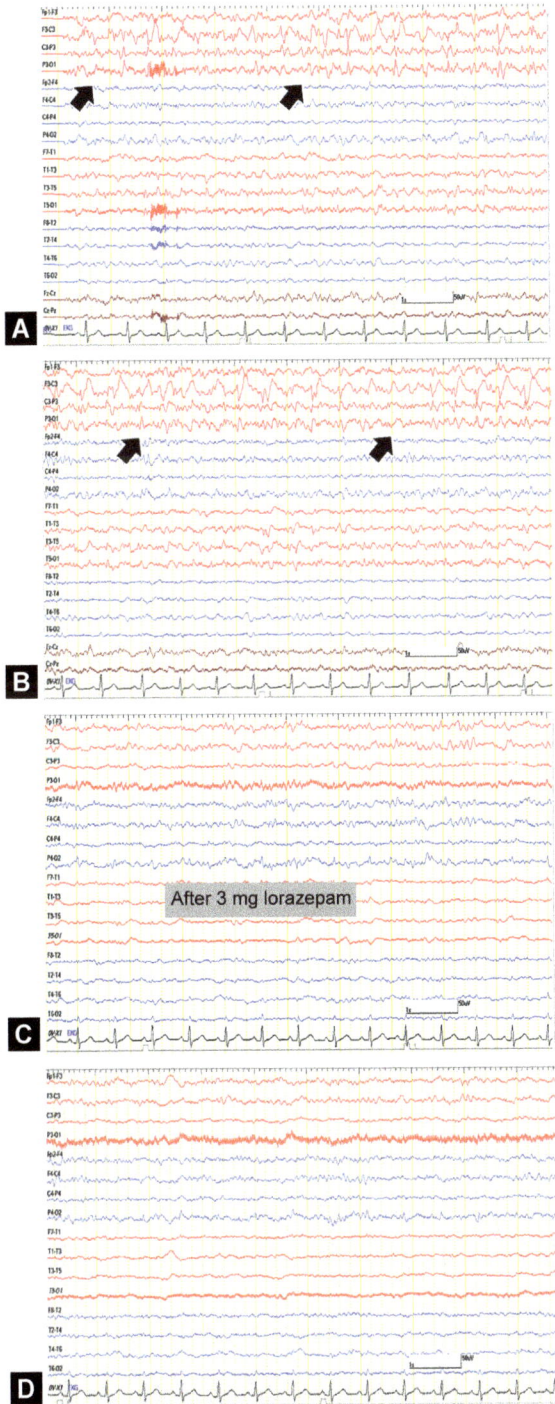

Figs. 2A to D: EEG showing rhythmic evolving ictal discharges (varying amplitude and voltage) at a frequency of 2.5–3 Hz marked in arrows diagnostic of focal NCSE. After administration of 3 mg of lorazepam EEG discharges disappeared (Benzodiazepine trial) followed by clinical response confirming the diagnosis of NCSE *(For color version, see Plate 3).*

With a possible exception of SE recovering to baseline, cEEG is mandatory and should be connected as early as possible.

Continuous EEG monitoring of patients up to 24 hours after clinical signs of SE had ended and revealed that nearly half of them continued to demonstrate electrographic seizures. EEG monitoring is an important tool in the management of SE. Higher mortality in SE was seen in patients with longer duration of CSE and in those with delay in diagnosis of NCSE. In resource-poor setting with limited availability of cEEG monitoring in countries such as India, at least frequent intermittent EEG should be done (at least twice a day) in the treatment of SE.

Investigations (Flowchart 2)

- Computed tomography (CT) and magnetic resonance imaging (MRI) brain for cause of SE
- *Lumbar puncture*:
  - For neuroinfections—viral, bacterial, tubercular, or fungal.
  - For autoimmune encephalitis [N-methyl-D-aspartate (NMDA), gamma-aminobutyric acid (GABA), α-amino-3-hydroxy-5-methyl-4-isoxazolepropionic acid (AMPA), anti-leucine-rich glioma inactivated-1 (LG1), contactin associated protein 2 (CASPR2), glutamic acid decarboxylase65 (GAD65)].

NONCONVULSIVE STATUS EPILEPTICUS

Nonconvulsive status epilepticus is an EEG diagnosis and is now increasingly being recognized in the intensive care unit (ICU) setting. A simple definition of NCSE is the alteration of consciousness or behavior from baseline state lasting for at least 30 minutes without convulsive movements, and with the presence of one or more of the following epileptiform patterns in the EEG:

- Repetitive focal or generalized epileptiform activity (spikes, sharp waves, spike-and-wave, and sharp-and-slow wave complexes) or rhythmic theta or delta activity at more than 3 per second.
- The above EEG changes at less than 3 per second, but with improvement or resolution of epileptic activity on EEG and improvement in the clinical state following intravenous (IV) injection of a rapidly acting AED, such as a benzodiazepine.
- A temporal evolution of epileptiform or rhythmic activity at more than 1 Hz with change in location or frequency over time.

Based on EEG, NCSE may be classified into focal and generalized NCSE. How aggressively one should treat NCSE in clinical practice is still debated. The clinician has to weigh the risks and benefits of aggressive treatment and

Flowchart 2: Algorithm for evaluation of status epilepticus.

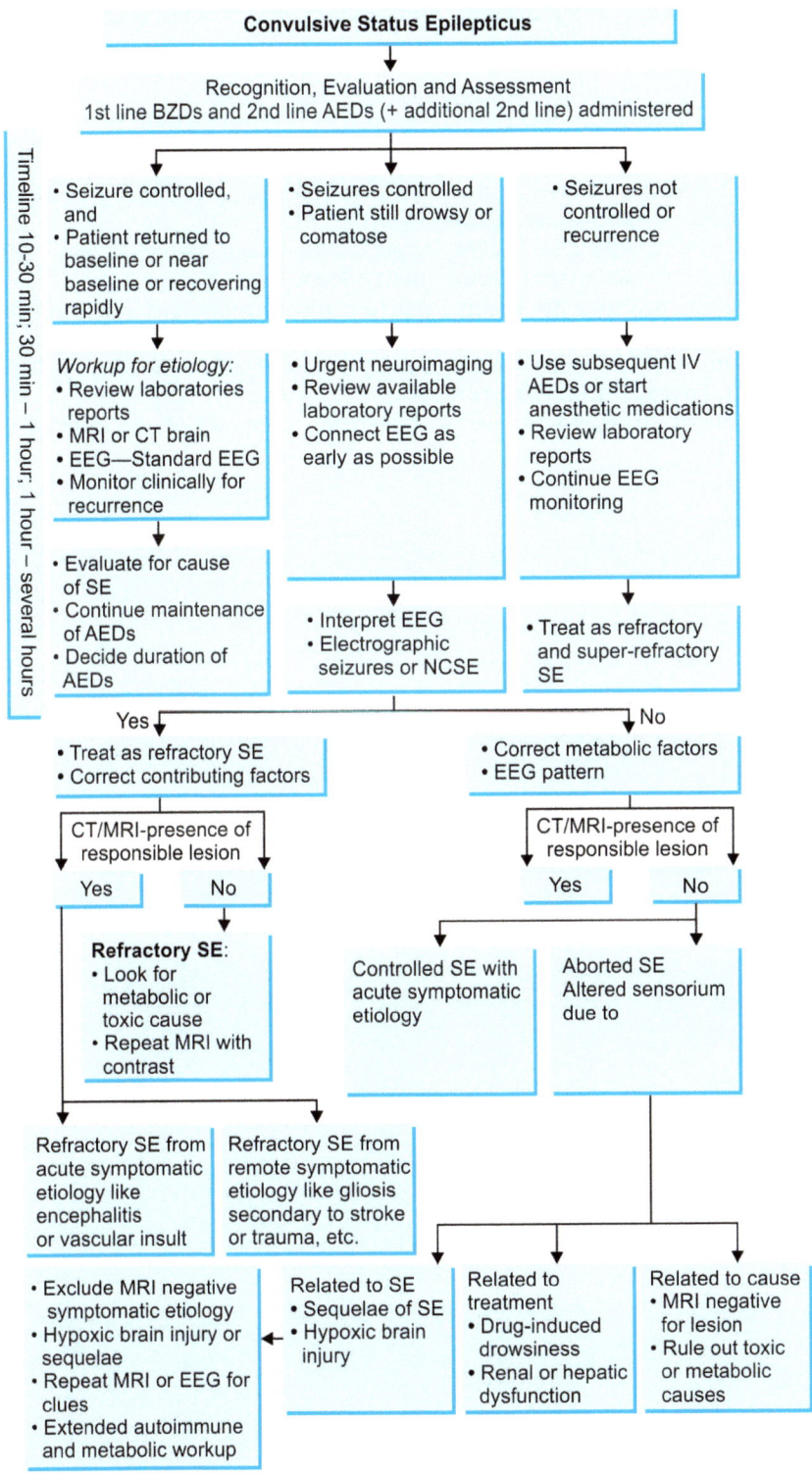

individualize treatment on case-to-case basis. Mortality in NCSE is determined by etiology, depth of coma, and development of acute complications and not by the nature of the EEG changes.

REFERENCES

1. Trinka E, Cock H, Hesdorffer D, et al. A definition and classification of status epilepticus—Report of the ILAE Task Force on Classification of Status Epilepticus. Epilepsia. 2015;56(10):1515-23.
2. Misra UK, Kalita J, Bhoi SK. Practice parameters in management of status epileptics. Ann Indian Acad Neurol. 2014;17(Suppl 1):S27-31.
3. Foreman B, Hirsch LJ. Epilepsy emergencies: diagnosis and management. Neurol Clin. 2012;30(1):11-41.
4. DeLorenzo RJ, Ko D, Towne AR, et al. Prediction of outcome in status epilepticus. Epilepsia. 1997;38(suppl 8):210-5.
5. Hantus S. Epilepsy emergencies. Continuum (Minneap Minn). 2016;22(1):173-90.

12 Drug Treatment: Choice of Antiepileptic Drugs

Sujit Kumar

INTRODUCTION

Epilepsy is a disorder known to mankind from time immemorial. The treatment of epilepsy requires not only a knowledge of antiepileptic drugs (AEDs) but a thorough understanding of the type of seizures, underlying syndrome, if any, etiological factors, age, gender, and associated medical comorbidity.

A systematic approach to medical treatment of epilepsy is outlined here. A detailed description of individual drugs and treatment in some special circumstances such as status epilepticus is beyond the purview of this chapter.

GOALS OF TREATMENT

The primary aim of drug treatment in epilepsy is to achieve seizure control with a good quality of life, with respect to medical improvement and other aspects of life. Complete seizure freedom with a reduction in adverse effects has been hailed to be the most consistent parameter associated with a good quality of life.[1]

Antiepileptic Drugs (AEDs): To Start or Not to Start

It is important to first confirm the diagnosis of a true seizure, attempt to establish the seizure type and syndrome, and select an AED on the basis of seizure type, spectrum of activity, tolerability, and drug interactions.

Single Unprovoked Seizure

A 30–40% risk of recurrence after a single unprovoked seizure has been noted in several studies. Factors, which put a patient at high risk for seizure recurrence, after a first seizure, include a neurological deficit at diagnosis, an abnormal magnetic resonance imaging (MRI) brain, an abnormal electroencephalography (EEG), and positive family history among first-degree relatives. AED therapy is recommended in these high risk patients as they have a better long-term outcome, in early versus delayed treatment.[2]

Two or More Unprovoked Seizures

There is a 73% risk of seizure recurrence within 4 years, for those with a history of two prior unprovoked seizures. The risk of a third seizure is nearly twofold higher in patients with remote symptomatic epilepsy than in those with genetic or no known cause. Drug therapy with AEDs is therefore recommended in those patients.[2]

AEDs: An Ideal Antiepileptic

The ideal AED would possess the "wish list" of the following properties—high efficacy, good tolerability, minimal drug interactions, simple administration schedules, as well as high-cost effectiveness. These properties are especially relevant when managing patients with combination therapy.[3]

AEDs: Strategies for Starting Therapy

The AED therapy remains the mainstay, achieving up to 70% seizure freedom in patients. As many as 50% of patients with newly diagnosed focal or generalized seizures, while taking the first appropriately selected and dosed first-line AED, will achieve seizure freedom. Hence, monotherapy is currently the best pharmacotherapeutic option and is being widely practiced, when first starting AED treatment.[3] An appropriate drug for the seizure type/syndrome should be selected by using an appropriate dosage and slowly titrated to optimal response (Box 1 and Table 1).

If monotherapy is poorly tolerated or ineffective, the strategy is to switch to another drug. If the first drug has partial efficacy and is well tolerated, it

Box 1: Preferred first-line antiepileptic drugs for new-onset epilepsy in adults.

New-onset partial epilepsies:
- Carbamazepine
- Levetiracetam
- Oxcarbazepine
- Topiramate
- Gabapentin
- Lamotrigine
- Valproate
- Phenytoin
- Phenobarbitone

New-onset idiopathic generalized epilepsies:
- Lamotrigine
- Valproate
- Levetiracetam
- Topiramate

Table 1: Dosages and suggested titration of antiepileptic drugs (AEDs).

AED	Suggested titration	Suggested range of average target dose (total mg/day); frequency of dosing
Carbamazepine	200 mg every 3 days	600–1,200 BID or TID
Clobazam	10–15 mg per day	10–40 mg BID
Eslicarbazepine	400 mg every 3–7 days	800–1,200
Felbamate	300 mg every 7 days	2,400–3,600 BID or TID
Lamotrigine	*Monotherapy:* 25 mg/2 week, 50 mg/2 week then increase frequency 50–100 mg/week. Add-on in the presence of valproate: 25 mg every other day for 2 week, 25 mg/day/2 week, then increases of 25–50 mg/week.	100–400 mg QID
Levetiracetam	500 mg every 1–3 days	1,000–3,000 BID
Oxcarbazepine	150 mg every 3–7 days	800–1,800 BID or TID
Phenobarbital	50 mg every 7 days	50–200 QD or BID
Phenytoin	50–100 mg every 3–5 days; beyond 200 mg in 25–30 mg steps	200–300 BID, TID, or QD for extended release availability
Retigabine	100 mg/day increased by 150 mg/day	900–1,200 BID or TID
Tiagabine	6 mg every 5–7 days	36–60 BID or TID
Topiramate	25 mg for 1–2 week; beyond 100 mg, 25–50 mg per week	100–400 BID or TID
Valproate	500 mg every 3–7 days	600–1,500 BID
Vigabatrin	500 mg every 7 days	500–3,000 BID

(BID: two times per day; QD: once a day; TID: three times per day)

is worth trying another drug in combination. Add-on therapy appears to be more effective when started immediately after first-drug failure, rather than after a second drug has also failed.[4] A rational approach might be to combine AEDs with different mechanisms, such as a sodium-channel blocker with an agent that enhances GABAergic inhibition.

AEDs: Choosing an AED

While starting monotherapy, a clear understanding of the seizure type, syndrome and patient characteristics, is imperative. Box 1 shows the preferred first-line antiepileptic drugs for new-onset and refractory epilepsy in adults.[2] Table 1 shows dosages of commonly used AEDs and suggested titration to achieve optimal response.[2]

While efficacy is an important consideration, avoidance of adverse effects is also important. Although complete seizure freedom is generally thought to be the most significant predictor of improved quality of life, adverse effects may be the most important negative influence on a person's perception of individual current health status.[1] Significant adverse events associated with established AEDs contribute to initial treatment failure in > 40% of patients (Table 2).[5]

Table 2: Adverse effects of antiepileptic drugs (AEDs).		
AED	Adverse effects	
	Neurological	Systemic
Phenytoin	Dizziness, diplopia, ataxia, incoordination, and confusion	Gum hyperplasia, lymphadenopathy, hirsutism, osteomalacia, facial coarsening, and skin rash
Carbamazepine	Ataxia, dizziness, diplopia, and vertigo	Aplastic anemia, leukopenia, gastrointestinal irritation, hepatotoxicity, and hyponatremia
Valproic acid	Ataxia, sedation, and tremor	Hepatotoxicity, thrombocytopenia, gastrointestinal irritation, weight gain, hyperammonemia, and transient alopecia
Lamotrigine	Dizziness, diplopia, sedation, ataxia, headache	Skin rash and Stevens-Johnson syndrome
Ethosuximide	Ataxia, lethargy, and headache	Skin rash, bone marrow depression, and gastrointestinal irritation
Topiramate	Psychomotor slowing, sedation, word finding difficulty, and fatigue paresthesias	Renal stones, hypohidrosis, weight loss, and glaucoma
Phenobarbitone	Sedation, ataxia, confusion, dizziness, decreased libido, and depression	Skin rash
Clobazam and clonazepam	Sedation, lethargy, and ataxia	Anorexia and sometimes weight gain
Felbamate	Insomnia, dizziness, sedation, and headache	Aplastic anemia, gastrointestinal irritation, hepatic failure, and weight loss
Levetiracetam	Sedation, fatigue, incoordination, behavioral changes, and psychosis	Anemia and leukopenia
Zonisamide	Sedation, headache, psychosis, dizziness, and confusion	Anorexia, hypohidrosis, renal stones, and weight loss
Oxcarbazepine	Dizziness, diplopia, vertigo, headache, and fatigue	Same as carbamazepine

General principle is "start low and go slow". Flexible titration to response and controlled dose escalation improve the tolerability of many drugs. If achieving seizure control is difficult, the maximum tolerated dose of the drug should be explored before adding the second drug, but a balance need to be achieved between adverse effects and seizure control.

AEDs: Pharmacokinetics

Pharmacokinetic drug interactions complicate management in patients on combination therapy or those receiving treatment for comorbid conditions, although dose adjustment and serum drug level monitoring (for some of the drugs) can overcome these problems. Toxicity may be increased and the efficacy of either the AEDs or the concomitant drugs reduced. Hepatic enzyme-inducing AEDs [e.g. carbamazepine (CBZ) and phenytoin (PHT)] have a high propensity for drug interactions. On the other hand, drug-drug interactions are unlikely with AEDs not metabolized by liver, notably gabapentin, levetiracetam, and topiramate.[3]

Hepatic enzyme-inducing AEDs may also affect the response to other drugs metabolized by similar pathways, e.g. warfarin, some tricyclic antidepressants, corticosteroids, some antineoplastic drugs, many antivirals, and cyclosporine. Conversely, fluoxetine, cimetidine, omeprazole, fluconazole, and erythromycin may increase the toxicity of hepatic enzyme-inducing AEDs.

AEDs: Therapeutic Monitoring

Phenytoin has nonlinear saturation dose kinetics and requires monitoring. However, monitoring of other AED plasma concentrations should be individualized to confirm suspected nonadherence or to evaluate suspected toxicity or uncontrolled seizures.[5]

AEDs: Stopping Antiepileptic Drugs in Patients on Remission

General principle is that after completion of 3–5 years of AED therapy, patients in remission may be tapered off AEDs. This decision, however, must be taken after a careful consideration of the type of epilepsy, clinical features, and in discussion with the patient and relatives.

Seizure freedom greater than 2 years implies a 60% chance of persistent remission in certain epilepsy syndromes. Other favorable factors for seizure remission on stopping AEDs include—control easily achieved on a low dose with one drug, no previous unsuccessful attempts at withdrawal, normal neurologic examination and EEG, and primary generalized epilepsy except juvenile myoclonic epilepsy and benign syndromes.

AEDs: Special Considerations

Age

Children with epilepsy have a more compromised quality of life in the psychological, social, and school domains. Some drugs such as levetiracetam, which exacerbate cognitive impairment and hyperactivity/behavioral issues in children and elderly, should be used with caution. The cognitive risk in many conditions (Lennox-Gastaut syndrome, West's syndrome, etc.) associated with severe epilepsy and encephalopathy is clearly reduced by AED treatment, provided it is chosen properly and administered early enough in the course of the disease.

As elderly patients are more likely to have comorbid conditions requiring combination therapy, drug interactions may be more frequent and adherence poorer. AEDs can also aggravate age-related cognitive deficits. In the elderly, drugs should be started at low doses to minimize adverse effects and drug interactions. Drug interactions are not only among AEDs but also with other drugs used for comorbid conditions.[3]

Women of Child-bearing Potential

Maternal and fetal risks associated with uncontrolled seizures have to be weighed against the increased risk of adverse outcomes in the offspring imposed by maternal use of AEDs during pregnancy. Despite the documented teratogenicity of AEDs and the scarce documentation of risks imposed by maternal seizures, uncontrolled tonic-clonic seizures present greater risks than drug therapy to the fetus, especially in late pregnancy. Hence, AEDs in optimal doses are indicated for the treatment of epilepsy during pregnancy, if this is considered necessary to control tonic–clonic seizures. The AEDs that have the lowest rates of malformations, such as lamotrigine, levetiracetam and oxcarbazepine, are often preferred for women with epilepsy who are contemplating pregnancy. The change in the treatment must be started prior to pregnancy. Also, the addition of folic acid prevents fetal malformations. In the third trimester of pregnancy, the dose of antiepileptics must be increased by one-third and can be reduced postpartum.[3]

Renal Failure

The clearance of AEDs that are eliminated completely (vigabatrin and gabapentin) or largely (primidone and topiramate) unchanged by the renal route will be reduced in these patients. This may necessitate dose adjustments, but it does not preclude the use of these AEDs in renal failure.

Liver Failure

Although many AEDs undergo hepatic metabolism, their clearance is seldom affected to an extent that it influences the risk to benefit ratio, except for severe hepatic failure. Valproate should be avoided, if possible, in patients with liver dysfunction due to its potential hepatotoxic effects. Phenobarbital and benzodiazepines should be avoided in advanced stages of hepatic failure because of the risk of induction or aggravation of hepatic encephalopathy.

Porphyria

The AEDs with hepatic enzyme-inducing potential should be avoided in patients with porphyria.

AEDs: Medically Refractory Epilepsy

Drug-resistant epilepsy may be defined as failure of adequate trials of two tolerated and appropriately chosen and used AED schedules (whether as monotherapies or in combination) to achieve sustained seizure freedom. About 30% of newly diagnosed epilepsies will become medically refractory. These patients have a poor quality of life with consequences on morbidity, quality of life, mortality, and social and cognitive function. These patients will benefit from treatment at a center specialized in management of medically refractory epilepsy and presurgical workup. Table 3 shows the drugs of choice in refractory epilepsies and their dosages/titration.

Proper treatment along with health education regarding epilepsy can be a beacon light to bring people with epilepsy out of the shadows and enable majority of them to lead a meaningful, happy, and productive life.

Table 3: The drugs of choice in refractory epilepsies and their dosages/titration.[2]		
Drugs for refractory epilepsies:		
Lacosamide	100 mg every 5–7 days	200–400 mg/day BID
Zonisamide TID Na	100 mg ever 3–7 days	200–600 BID
Clobazam	10 mg per day	10–40 mg BID or QD
Perampanel	2 mg every 3–7 days	8–12 QD
Brivaracetam	50 mg every 5–7 days	100–200 mg BID

(BID: two times a day; QD: once a day; TID: three times a day)

REFERENCES

1. Birbeck GL, Hays RD, Cui X, et al. Seizure reduction and quality-of-life improvements in people with epilepsy. Epilepsia. 2002;43(5):535-8.
2. Schmidt D. Starting, choosing, changing and discontinuing drug treatment for epilepsy patients. Neurol Clin. 2016;34(2):363-81.
3. Sander JW. The use of antiepileptic drugs—principles and practice. Epilepsia. 2004;45(Suppl. 6):28-34.
4. Kwan P, Brodie MJ. Epilepsy after the first drug fails: substitution or add-on? Seizure. 2000;9(7): 464-8.
5. Greenwood RS. Adverse effects of antiepileptic drugs. Epilepsia. 2000;41(Suppl. 2):S42-52.

13
Diagnosis of Epilepsy

Sarma GRK

INTRODUCTION

Seizures and epilepsies are common neurological problems that are managed by physicians both in the emergency department and in routine practice. A diagnosis of epilepsy is best achieved by a thoroughly elicited history, review of home videos, if available, meticulous observation during a seizure, and further supported by neuroimaging and electroencephalogram (EEG). Since a significant proportion of neuroimaging and EEGs turn out to be inconclusive, clinical data still forms the backbone of epilepsy diagnosis and classification.

The internationally accepted terminologies and classification of these conditions have been undergoing constant revision and refinement, necessitating a periodic update for the physicians. This chapter addresses these issues in the light of the new International League against Epilepsy (ILAE) Classification of Seizures and Epilepsies (2017), which provides a useful framework. Classifying the patient's epilepsy to a particular category serves many purposes. It suggests possible etiologies, expected course and prognosis, and choice of antiepileptic drugs, and it predicts cognitive-psychiatric dysfunction and, sometimes, the genetic factors. The ILAE acknowledges that the current classification is based on a combination of expert opinion and scientific evidence, as the latter is not advanced enough today to provide a purely scientific and rigorous classification. Diagnosis and classification of epilepsy in a given patient is a multilevel framework (Fig. 1) that includes:
- *Level 1*: Identification of seizure type
- *Level 2*: Identification of epilepsy type
- *Level 3*: Identification of epilepsy syndrome
- At all levels, etiology must be sought and mentioned
- At all levels, comorbidities must be identified and mentioned.

LEVEL 1: IDENTIFICATION OF SEIZURE TYPE

A seizure is defined as "a transient occurrence of signs and/or symptoms due to abnormal excessive or synchronous neuronal activity in the brain".

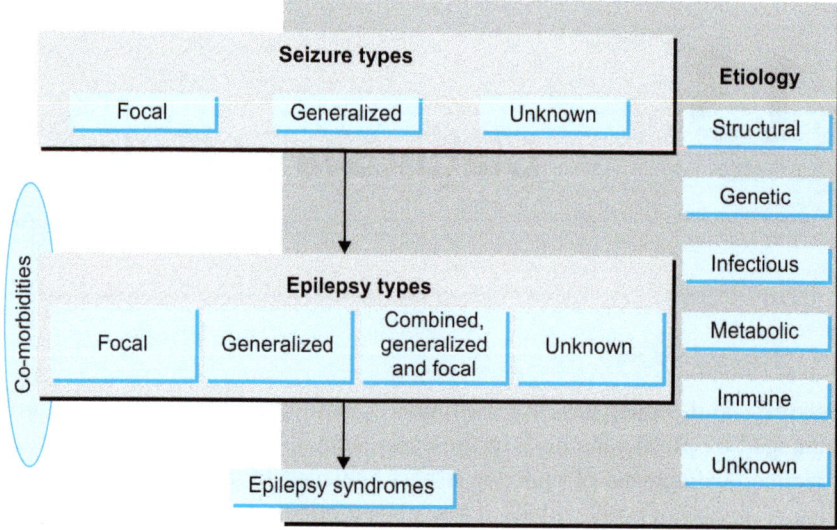

Fig. 1: The International League against Epilepsy (ILAE) framework for classification of epilepsies.

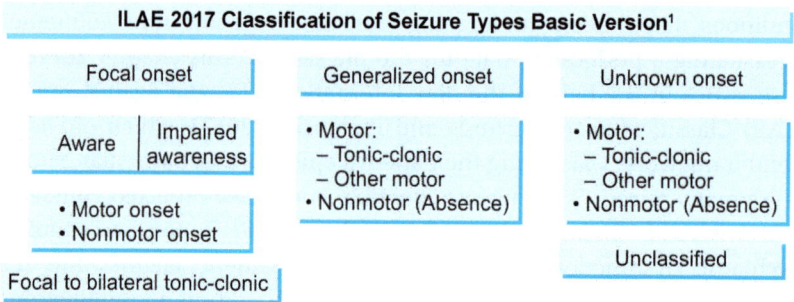

Fig. 2: International League against Epilepsy (ILAE) 2017 classification of seizure types basic version.

The clinician must ensure first that the patient has a true epileptic seizure and not one of its mimics such as syncope or psychogenic events. The next step is classification into a seizure type according to the ILAE seizure type classification (2017). The taskforce provided a basic version (Fig. 2) and also an expanded version, either of which may be used depending on the clinician's level of confidence in characterizing the seizure type.

It begins with determination of whether the onset is focal or generalized or unknown. A focal seizure may be associated with preserved awareness (the person is aware of self and environment even if immobile). In contrast, in a focal impaired awareness seizure (equivalent to "complex partial seizure" in the previous classification), the person is unaware of self and environment. In addition, the focal seizure may be classified as "motor" or "nonmotor" depending on the predominant manifestation. Focal seizures may be further classified by the predominant earliest component of the seizure into various motor (tonic, clonic, myoclonic, atonic, hyperkinetic, automatisms, and epileptic spasms) or nonmotor subtypes (somatosensory, visual, auditory, autonomic, cognitive, emotional, or behavior arrest). When a seizure has a focal onset but progresses to bilateral convulsive movements, it is called focal to bilateral tonic-clonic seizure (previously "partial onset with secondary generalized seizure").

The term "generalized" implies that a seizure involves bilateral (not necessarily "all") networks from the onset. Generalized seizures can also be motor (tonic-clonic, tonic, clonic, myoclonic, atonic, or epileptic spasms) or nonmotor (absence seizures—typical or atypical/myoclonic absences). They may be asymmetrical, causing difficulties in differentiating from focal seizures. In a significant proportion of seizures, the onset cannot be ascertained with confidence due lack of reliable eye witness account. Such seizures have to be classified as "unknown onset seizures" until more information is available during follow-up.

LEVEL 2: IDENTIFICATION OF EPILEPSY TYPE

Epilepsy was defined conceptually in 2005 as a disorder of the brain characterized by an enduring predisposition to generate epileptic seizures. Previous practical definitions required occurrence of at least 2 unprovoked seizures more than 24 hours apart. In a major shift from this notion, the current classification (2014, ILAE) accepts the diagnosis of epilepsy even after a single unprovoked or reflex seizure, if one of the following conditions is fulfilled:

- A probability of further seizures similar to the general recurrence risk (>60%), after two unprovoked seizures, occurring over the next 10 years, (example: single seizure occurring more than a week after a stroke)
  Or
- A diagnosis of an epilepsy syndrome.

  Once the diagnosis of "epilepsy" is accepted, it may be placed in one of the four categories:
  1. *Focal epilepsy*: The diagnosis is made on clinical grounds (focal seizure semiology) supported by focal epileptiform discharges in EEG (which may not be present in a significant proportion of cases).
  2. *Generalized epilepsy*: The diagnosis is made again on clinical grounds (generalized seizures) supported by generalized epileptiform discharges in EEG. If the EEG is normal, one cannot be certain of

"generalized epilepsy" unless there is a family history of generalized epilepsy or there is occurrence of myoclonic jerks that point to a specific syndrome like juvenile myoclonic epilepsy (JME).
3. *Generalized and focal epilepsy*: This new category is created to accommodate disorders such as Lennox-Gastaut syndrome in which both focal and generalized seizures and EEG changes can occur. These are usually difficult to treat epilepsies associated with significant cognitive impairment and need to be referred to a neurologist or an epileptologist.
4. *Unknown*: Often, the seizure type and epilepsy type cannot be determined due to inadequate clinical and EEG data. In such situations, the epilepsy is classified as "unknown" type until further clarity emerges.

LEVEL 3: IDENTIFICATION OF EPILEPSY SYNDROME

An epilepsy syndrome refers to a cluster of features incorporating seizure types, EEG, and imaging features that tend to occur together. A syndrome usually has a distinctive clinical course, prognosis, comorbidities, treatment response, and often etiological implications. The ILAE does not offer any formal classification of epilepsy syndromes. Some important generalized and focal epilepsy syndromes in clinical practice are shown in Table 1.

Some changes in terminologies may be noted. The generalized epilepsy syndromes have earlier been termed "idiopathic generalized epilepsies (IGE)", whereas the new term "genetic generalized epilepsy (GGE)" is used when there is reasonable evidence and confidence exists to invoke a genetic etiology. The disadvantage of the term "genetic generalized epilepsy" is the risk of confusion between "genetic" and "inherited" disease in the lay public and its social and marital implications. Hence, the term "IGE" may still be used in clinical practice. Some age-dependent focal epilepsies were earlier termed "benign" and are now called "self-limited" focal epilepsies because of the recognition that the outcomes, especially cognitive behavioral, may not always be benign. Similarly, the terms "catastrophic" and "malignant" have been abandoned.

Table 1: Some important epilepsy syndromes.

Generalized	Focal

• Childhood absence epilepsy
• Juvenile absence epilepsy
• Juvenile myoclonic epilepsy, and
• Generalized tonic-clonic seizures alone
	• Self-limited epilepsy with centrotemporal spikes
	• Self-limited occipital epilepsies of childhood:
	  – Early-onset form (Panayiotopoulos type)
	  – Late-onset form (Gastaut type)

ETIOLOGY

The clinician should make every effort to identify the etiology of epilepsy, which may belong to one of the six major categories (Fig. 1). The etiologies are not hierarchical or mutually exclusive: a patient may have a structural lesion due to a genetic abnormality (example is cortical tuber due to tuberin mutation), in which case he has both structural and genetic etiology. Similarly, patients with tuberculoma and seizures are considered to have infection related and structural etiology. Common examples of various etiological groups are listed below:

- *Structural etiology*: Trauma, stroke, tumor, malformations, infections, hippocampal sclerosis, and gliosis.
- *Genetic etiology*: *KCNQ1* mutation causing benign neonatal familial convulsions, unknown mutation causing autosomal-dominant nocturnal frontal lobe epilepsy, *SCNA1* mutation causing Dravet syndrome, etc.
- *Infectious etiology*: Epilepsy due to infectious etiology must be differentiated from acute symptomatic seizures during an active infection like meningoencephalitis. Common infectious causes of epilepsy, worldwide, are cysticercosis, tuberculosis, cerebral malaria, toxoplasmosis, and congenital TORCH infections.
- *Metabolic etiology*: It includes conditions with well-delineated metabolic defect with epilepsy as one of the clinical features. Examples include pyridoxine-dependent seizures, aminoacidopathies, and porphyria. Again, acute symptomatic seizures due to metabolic derangements such as hyponatremia are not to be called "metabolic epilepsies".
- *Immune etiology*: It represents epilepsy due to autoimmune-mediated central nervous system inflammation. Examples include anti-NMDA (N-methyl-D-aspartate) receptor encephalitis and anti-LGI1 (Leucine-rich glioma-inactivated 1) encephalitis.
- *Unknown etiology*: When the exact etiology of epilepsy is not yet established, it is placed in this category.

COMORBIDITIES

A number of comorbidities are being increasingly recognized even in the so-called "benign" epilepsies and are listed below. An early identification and management of these are important to improve the quality of life of persons with epilepsy.

- Learning disability
- Behavioral problems
- Psychiatric conditions
- Sleep disorders
- Motor disabilities
- Movement disorders
- Gait problems.

INVESTIGATION OF EPILEPSY

Electroencephalography

Electroencephalography (EEG) is a commonly ordered investigation, but a clinician must understand its exact role and limitations in the diagnosis of epilepsy. A standard EEG is performed by applying 16 surface electrodes on standard points of scalp (10-20 international system of lead placement) and recording that lasts at least 20-30 minutes. Various activation procedures such as hyperventilation, photic stimulation, and spontaneous sleep are utilized to increase the yield.

- Absence of epileptiform discharges (EDs) does not exclude the diagnosis of epilepsy, as the sensitivity of first EEG in epilepsy is only 25-50%. The sensitivity increases up to 90% by repeated or prolonged recordings.
- If the epileptogenic zone is located in mesial or basal cortical regions, no EDs may be recorded on surface electrodes. This may result in false-negative diagnosis in a patient with epilepsy.
- Specificity of EEG in diagnosis of epilepsy is 78-98%. Thus, presence of EDs does not necessarily confirm the diagnosis of epilepsy. As an example, only 40% of children with centrotemporal spikes have epilepsy. About 0.5% of apparently healthy persons have EDs on EEG. 20-30% of patients with structural lesions such as tumors and head injuries may have EDs without clinical seizures.
- Several benign discharges are often misdiagnosed as EDs by EEG readers resulting in false-positive diagnosis of epilepsy. Such misleading nonepileptiform activities include vertex sharp waves and K-complexes of sleep, benign epileptiform transients of sleep (BETS), wicket spikes, positive occipital sharp transients of sleep (POSTS), etc.
- Some EEG patterns have strong correlation with a particular epilepsy syndrome. For example, 3 Hz generalized spike wave discharges in absence epilepsy, hypsarrhythmia in infantile spasms.
- A properly performed and interpreted EEG helps in the multiaxial diagnosis of epilepsy (focal versus generalized, or a specific epilepsy syndrome). This may guide appropriate antiepileptic drug selection.

Neuroimaging in the Diagnosis of Epilepsy

Computed tomography (CT) scan and magnetic resonance imaging (MRI) are the two important imaging techniques in the initial evaluation of epilepsy and will be discussed further. Functional imaging and newer MRI techniques are typically used in evaluation of refractory epilepsy and will not be discussed here.

- Neuroimaging is warranted in most patients with epilepsy. Some exceptions are benign neonatal myoclonic epilepsy and typical absence epilepsy.
- If a patient has highly recurrent seizures, focal deficits, progressive cognitive decline, altered sensorium, headache, fever, papilledema, or history of head trauma, an emergency imaging is warranted.
- Overall, MRI has higher yield than CT scan in epilepsy and must be considered the imaging modality of first choice. A CT scan scores over MRI, if patient is uncooperative or has a contraindication for MRI or in acute head injury. Calcifications, hemorrhages, and bone lesions are more easily appreciated on CT scan. Economic factor and availability are important determinants in resource-poor settings.
- 1.5-Tesla MRI is adequate for most clinical situations. 3-Tesla MRI with specific epilepsy protocols is utilized in epilepsy centers as a part of presurgical evaluation of refractory epilepsy.
- A normal MRI does not exclude a structural cause of epilepsy. For example, small cortical dysplasias are difficult to appreciate on standard MRI.
- Presence of an MRI lesion does not prove it to be the cause of epilepsy. For example, mesial temporal sclerosis may be seen in some nonepileptic persons. Hence, the MRI lesion must be correlated with clinical and EEG data to ascertain the epileptogenic potential of the lesion.
- A number of well-known epileptogenic lesions can be clearly demonstrated on MRI. These include focal cortical dysplasias, tuberous sclerosis, cavernous angioma, neurodevelopmental tumors, Sturge–Weber syndrome, Rasmussen encephalitis, gliotic lesions, cysticercal granulomas, congenital malformations, hypothalamic hamartomas, and a variety of brain tumors.
- A radiologist, experienced in neuroimaging, makes a crucial difference in improving the yield of MRI in epilepsy.

Laboratory Investigations

Hemogram and biochemical tests can reveal a medical condition as a cause of seizures. Such conditions include diabetes, uremia, hypothyroidism, hypoparathyroidism, dyselectrolytemia, and chronic liver disease. In appropriate setting, serology for syphilis, HIV, workup for collagen vascular disorders, and autoimmune and paraneoplastic syndromes is warranted. In a patient with clear dysmorphic features or strong family history of epilepsy, a geneticist opinion may clinch the diagnosis.

SUGGESTED READING

1. Cendes F, Theodore WH, Brinkmann BH, et al. Neuroimaging of epilepsy. Handb Clin Neurol. 2016;136:985-1014.

2. Fisher RS, Cross JH, French JA, et al. Operational classification of seizure types by the International League Against Epilepsy: Position Paper of the ILAE Commission for Classification and Terminology. Epilepsia. 2017;58(4):522-30.
3. Scheffer IE, Berkovic S, Capovilla G, et al. ILAE classification of the epilepsies: Position paper of the ILAE Commission for Classification and Terminology. Epilepsia. 2017;58(4):512-21.
4. Smith SJM. EEG in the diagnosis, classification and management of patients with epilepsy. J Neurol Neurosurg Psychiatr. 2005;76 (Suppl II):ii2-ii7.

14 Drug Withdrawal after Seizure Freedom: When and How?

Rai PV

INTRODUCTION

Drug treatment of epileptic seizures is the first line of epilepsy management, which is usually a long-term procedure. Hence, initiation of drugs after the diagnosis of epilepsy based mostly on the occurrence of two unprovoked seizures and later withdrawal of drugs after a seizure freedom of 2–5 years must be done carefully considering the medical and social aspects of the person with epilepsy (PWE). Regarding the initiation of drugs, there is some consensus, which is not the case, related to drug withdrawal. Factors related to the age of seizure onset, types of epilepsy related to idiopathic, symptomatic, epileptic syndromes of childhood and adults, as well as prognosis of the individual epilepsy must be taken fully into consideration before taking a decision to withdraw the drugs. Equally important are the social aspects of the PWE and his or her motivation for the withdrawal of drugs. These factors must be considered irrespective of the duration of seizure freedom.

The diagnosis of epilepsy is rather a serious event in the life of any person. After the initial diagnosis, practically every one is advised to take antiepileptic drugs (AEDs), which is a long-term procedure. The frequent questions asked by patients and relatives are: Is my epilepsy permanent? How long the drugs should be taken? What are the side effects? There are no standard answers to these questions because of several medical and individual factors.

However, the clinician must make every attempt to give acceptable answers based on the available evidence. Whatever is said at this stage carries much importance regarding the further patient compliance.

In the clinical practice, one experiences generally two types of PWE. After initial disappointment, most people accept epilepsy diagnosis (or any other long-term disease) as destiny and the long-term drugs as an "unpleasant necessity". Such persons remain committed to the regular intake of drugs. There are others, rather a minority, who have difficulty to accept the diagnosis of epilepsy and search all possible literature and personal examples to disapprove the diagnosis. Such people when confronted with the necessity of medication have even more problems to take regular drugs and seek help with different alternative therapies. It depends on the convincing art of the clinician to mobilize cooperation of such patients.

Since the advent of first four AEDs—phenobarbitone (PB), phenytoin (PHT), carbamazepine (CBZ), and sodium valproate (VPT)—success of seizure control has reached around 70%. Further drugs have contributed for better management of epilepsies with reduction of side effects and improvement of quality of life.

Based on several studies, it has become a common practice to start AED after the occurrence of two unprovoked seizures, which is the present day criterion for epilepsy diagnosis.[1-3] Recent classification of epilepsy by International League against Epilepsy (ILAE), 2017 considers the diagnosis of epilepsy even after the first unprovoked epileptic seizure under certain conditions. The reason for doing this is the increased risk of further seizures without medication. With diagnosis/differential diagnosis of seizures and type of epilepsy and under proper drug selection, almost 80% reach remission, early after introduction of the drug.[2] Still, it is not clear whether these people have a considerably better prognosis of remaining free of seizures after later withdrawal of drugs. In spite of several studies over the decades, there is also no proper consensus as to how many years after seizure freedom under medication, the drugs can be withdrawn without the risk of seizure recurrence. There is some general understanding that careful withdrawal of drugs should be considered for children after 1-3 years of seizure remission and for adults after 3-5 years.[3] However, various clinical and social aspects must be considered before attempting to withdraw medication even in people with favorable prognosis because of the risk of relapse.

BENEFITS OF DRUG WITHDRAWAL

Epilepsy is not only a very common neurological disease but one which has very good chances of treatment, thanks to the present day availability of wide spectrum of AEDs. Some PWE become free of seizures under a single drug fairly fast after drug initiation and continue to remain seizure free. Some of these epilepsies have been identified as idiopathic epilepsies with isolated generalized tonic-clonic seizures (GTCS) in otherwise healthy children and young adults. Persons with absences starting in school age have a good prognosis and correspondingly become early free of seizures under medication. Even though these people generally are favorable candidates for later drug withdrawal, there are some marked exceptions as in the case juvenile myoclonic epilepsy (JME) where the rate of relapse is very high and hence requires almost lifelong treatment.

In the event of good seizure remission under drugs, it still becomes difficult for the clinician to decide whether and where the remission is a "cure" and where it is only a "control" with drugs. However, a PWE has clear advantages when the drug is withdrawn after longer remission of seizures not only in view of the side effects but also from the point of view of social stigma. Continued intake of drugs can be a handicap for a young person, for example when going to partnership/getting married or in the professional sphere, and the stoppage of drugs would mean "cure" and a feeling of freedom. Further, even under low medication, some long-term cognitive side effects cannot be ruled out. In young women planning pregnancy, drug withdrawal removes the fear of teratogenic side effects.[4,5]

RISKS OF DRUG WITHDRAWAL

Epileptic seizure with or without drugs is a major medical and social problem. Control of seizures, therefore, is the primary requisite. Quality of life improves considerably for a PWE after the remission of seizures even under medication. Studies, however, show that there is 20% recurrence of seizures after drug withdrawal in children and 40% recurrence in adults.[1,2] Not much clear data is available regarding the recurrence of seizures in PWE who continue to take drugs after remission of seizures even after period of 3-5 years, it is considered clearly lower. We still do not know the proper mechanisms of seizure control under AEDs, although quite some information is available regarding the different channels of drug action such as sodium, calcium, and GABA. It is also not always clear why a single epileptic seizure remains isolated and further seizures lead to the diagnosis of epilepsy. One possible explanation is based on the old concept of William Gowers that "Seizure begets Seizure", which means that every seizure may create a certain dysfunction in the neuronal activity and be the cause for further seizures. It can be presumed that AEDs through their mode of action are in a position to "heal" this dysfunction and lead to the process of cure or control seizures permanently as the case may be. However, it is difficult to assess this situation clinically, hence, attempts must be made to get data from the clinical studies for the purpose of practical management related to drug withdrawal.

CONDITIONS FAVORABLE FOR DRUG WITHDRAWAL

- Preferably 2-3 years of seizure remission for children and 3-5 years of remission for adults.
- Idiopathic generalized epilepsy with single kind of seizures, e.g. GTCS and/or absences.
- Only a small number of seizures and short duration of epilepsy before reaching remission under drug therapy.
- Normal electroencephalography (EEG) findings during the seizure-free period (for generalized epilepsies).

- No neurological deficits/normal MRI findings.
- Monotherapy of AEDs.
- Motivation of PWE and relatives.
- Not dependent on driving or working on heavy machines (for professional purpose).

CONDITIONS UNFAVORABLE FOR DRUG WITHDRAWAL

- Multiple seizures, focal epilepsy, and JME.
- Longer duration for seizure freedom after the introduction of AEDs.
- Longer duration of epilepsy.
- Positive family history among first-degree relatives (genetic epilepsy).
- Presence of neurological deficits.
- Abnormal EEG/MRI findings even after seizure freedom.
- Lesser motivation of PWE/relatives in view of drug withdrawal.
- Necessity of driving or working on heavy machines (for professional purpose).
- Multiple drug therapy needed to reach seizure remission.

PROGNOSIS AFTER DRUG WITHDRAWAL

Several studies are available as follow-up after the withdrawal of drugs,[5] some of them also in comparison with patients taking drugs after remission of seizures for 2–3 years. In a major study by the American Academy of Neurology (AAN),[4] 1,013 patients were randomized after 2 years seizure freedom and after the drugs withdrawal. After 2 years of follow-up, the patients with drug withdrawal had 41% relapse, whereas patients on drugs had 22% relapse.

The peak of relapse for withdrawal group was at 9 months. After further 2 years of follow-up of both groups, this scenario changed that at the end of 4 years, there was no significant difference in the relapse rate of patients under drugs and those where drugs were withdrawn.[4,5]

In the clinical practice, this is an indicator that attempts must be made to withdraw AEDs after a seizure-free period of 2–5 years although under individual considerations.

PRACTICAL GUIDELINES FOR DRUG WITHDRAWAL

- It is advisable to tell every patient/relative, even under favorable conditions, that a complete seizure-free period of 2–3 years for children and 3–5 years for adults under drug therapy may be necessary for drug withdrawal.
- The PWE should be free of all kinds of seizure even "small ones" history taking from relatives is useful.

- The tapering of drugs should be done very slowly over a period of 6 months to 1 year, the patient compliance is needed.
- A unit of drug, for example, PB—30 mg, PHT—50 mg, CBZ—100 mg, and VPT—200 mg, levetiracetam—250 mg, lamotrigine—50 mg, can be reduced every 2-3 months under clinical observation.
- It is useful to do at least one standard EEG after the reduction of about 50% of drugs.
- Person with epilepsy/relatives should be informed about possible risk of relapse, if they are unwilling to take the risk, the procedure should not be carried out.
- The PWE should avoid driving a vehicle or working on heavy machines during the procedure of drug withdrawal.

From different studies,[1,2] the recurrence of seizures is reported about 6 months after complete drug tapering. It is difficult to interpret the relapse either as a "withdrawal seizure" or as "reactivation" of epilepsy. Further procedure of eventual reintroduction of drug or waiting without drug must be decided after complete approval of the patient/relative.

Considering various studies available up to date, the clinician has a responsibility to try withdrawal of antiepileptic drugs in PWE after a seizure-free period of globally 2-5 years, in spite of the risk of recurrence of seizures.[2,4] As mentioned, motivation should come from patients/relatives, but the clinician could take the initiative of motivating the patient wherever possible. There are some extreme situations, however, which have to be handled with caution. The following two case histories belong to rather such extreme cases.

Case History 1

A female patient in Germany in the late 1970s. During the treatment, she was around 60 years of age. At the age of 40, she had in the history 3-5 GTCS about 1 hour after awakening. After the first three seizures, she received a medication of PB 100 mg per day. She had probably one or two more seizures soon after that but remained free of seizures for many years, certainly not less than 15 years.

After some initial tiredness, the patient had no side effects or any other complaints. She was an educated person and working part time. She had no neurological or psychological deficits but by nature somewhat anxious person. Her EEG showed rarely a short spike wave activity only during hyperventilation, over the years even this activity disappeared. The serum level for PB was rather low. The patient was a married woman and had an adult daughter who was a social worker in an epilepsy center.

Under the initiative of the daughter, the patient was brought for withdrawal of AED after a seizure freedom of 15 years. The patient totally refused the withdrawal for fear of relapse. Counseling did not help. The daughter brought the patient again after 3 years, now with 18 years of seizure freedom.

This time after much counseling, the patient agreed for partial withdrawal of drug. A plan was made for reduction of PB each unit of 25 mg to be reduced in an unusually long interval of every 3 months. After the first 3 months, an EEG was done, which was normal, also under hyperventilation. The second consultation happened after 6 months under similar conditions. The patient was becoming visibly anxious and refused to accept further withdrawal, after 75 mg of PB was withdrawn after a period of 9 months. She predicted that she would get a seizure, if PB was further reduced. The serum level for PB was very low and the EEG again normal, with further convincing through the daughter and clinician, the PB was withdrawn after 1 year of tapering and almost 20 years of seizure freedom.

Around 8 weeks after the withdrawal of last dosage of PB, the patient had a GTCS about 1 hour after awakening at home making her prediction come true. This happened most probably because of long period of anxiety and sleep deprivation. Hence, the seizure must be considered as a withdrawal seizure as well as provoked due to the reasons mentioned above and probably had no further consequences. However, the patient started taking 50 mg of PB immediately after the seizure. This could also be idiopathic generalized epilepsy with genetic component, which might need even longer treatment.

Case History 2

A female patient in Switzerland in the 1980s. At the time of treatment, she was about 45 years of age; she was highly educated person and having a very responsible social position. She was married and had no children. In the history at the age of 40, she had 2-3 GTCS in sleep in intervals of 3-4 weeks, the seizures were noticed by her husband. She would get the seizures out of deep sleep and would sleep further; and in one of the seizures, she had a tongue bite otherwise some muscle pain next morning; she was not convinced that the seizures were epileptic but the description of the husband was clear for GTCS. The patient had a complete medical examination at a renowned epilepsy clinic in USA. All the findings including clinical neurological, EEG in sleep, and MRI were normal. The patient was advised AED, had much reservation to take a drug. The selection of drug was also difficult as there was no clarity about the type of epilepsy excepting "sleep epilepsy". VPT, PHT, and PB were found unsuitable. The probable diagnosis was some kind of cryptogenic epilepsy. CBZ was given in a slowly increasing dosage of 200 mg 1-0-1. After the initiation of the drug, the patient became free of seizures. She was not happy of the drug intake complained about side effects. After 1 year of seizure freedom, she approached me for withdrawal of CBZ, which I declined.

After seizure freedom of 2 years, she approached again and insisted on drug withdrawal. EEG and other findings were normal. A plan was made to withdraw each unit of 50 mg of CBZ at an interval of 3 months. She was seen under a daily dosage of 350 mg of CBZ and was doing well. After 6 months, she was taking 300 mg of CBZ per day, after 9 months, she reached a dosage of 250 mg of CBZ per day. Three weeks under this dosage, she reacted with a GTCS at night, which she did not accept but was reported by the husband.

Two weeks later, she had a second GTCS in sleep. With much persuasion, the dosage of CBZ was raised to 300 mg per day and under this dosage, she remained free of seizures for 1 year and came again for further withdrawal of drug.

A second attempt was made to reduce the drug again with units of 50 mg of CBZ. This time she had a GTCS in sleep a month after the reduction of dosage to 250 mg per day and one more seizure, which followed just a few days later. All the neurological findings were again normal. The drug dosage was raised to 300 mg, which made the patient free of seizures. This is probably a case where the seizure is not a withdrawal seizure but it is epilepsy, which needs long-term medication, even though the dosage required was rather low. This shows that some patients become free of seizures on a low dosage of AEDs, without which, however, they tend to relapse of seizures.

REFERENCES

1. David C. Social Implications of Drug Treatment and Withdrawal. In: Ross E, Chadwick D, Crawford R (Eds). Epilepsy in Young People. USA: John Wiley & Sons Ltd; 1987.
2. Annegers JF, Hauser WA, Elveback LR. Remission in Seizures and relapse in patients with epilepsy. Epilepsia. 1979;20(6):729-37.
3. Srinivas HV. Manuel of Epilepsy. New Delhi: Jaypee Brothers Medical Publishers (P) Ltd.; 2016. pp. 49-50.
4. Hixon JD. Stopping antiepileptic drugs: when and why? Curr Treat Options Neurol. 2010;12(5):434-42.
5. Sirven JI, Sperling M, Wingerchuk DM. Early versus late antiepileptic drug withdrawal for people with epilepsy in remission. Cochrane Data Base Syst Rev. 2001;(3):CD001902.

15

Therapy Resistance and Management

Ravindranadh Chowdary M

INTRODUCTION

Therapy resistance in epilepsy is not uncommon and it is frustrating to the patient, caregivers, and to the treating physicians. Though it is a difficult problem, with careful and focused evaluation, we can help most of the patients by appropriate management.

Physicians need to be updated and aware about the possible treatment options available to this subset of patients. In this chapter, required approach for therapy resistance by physicians will be discussed.

DEFINITION AND ITS EVALUATION

There is no ideal definition for refractory epilepsy. Before the ILAE consensus definition (2009), different studies used different definitions. This led to difficulty in interpreting the results of various studies. Berg and Kelly[1] reviewed this problem in their study in 2006 and emphasized the need for the development of uniform consensus definition. In 2010, the ILAE taskforce proposed the new definition of drug-resistant epilepsy (DRE) as "failure of adequate trials of two tolerated and appropriately chosen and used antiepileptic drug (AED) schedules (whether as monotherapies or in combination) to achieve sustained seizure freedom".[2]

EPIDEMIOLOGY

It is estimated, in various studies, that the overall prevalence of epilepsy in India is 5.59–10 per 1,000.[3] About one-third of the newly diagnosed patients with epilepsy will be drug resistant.[4]

ETIOPATHOGENESIS AND PREDICTORS OF REFRACTORY EPILEPSY

The etiology of refractory epilepsy can be idiopathic (genetic), symptomatic, or cryptogenic. Idiopathic generalized epilepsies [childhood absence epilepsy/juvenile myoclonic epilepsy (JME)/ juvenile absence epilepsy (JAE)] can be relatively well controlled. About 7–10% of DRE patients constitute idiopathic generalized epilepsy.[5,6] About 80% of refractory epilepsies are due to symptomatic causes,[5,6] which include mesial temporal sclerosis, focal cortical dysplasia, calcified foci, post-traumatic gliosis, developmental tumors, and old stroke with gliosis. A subset of refractory epilepsy patients, especially type-1 focal cortical dysplasia, is MR negative.

The exact pathophysiology of refractory epilepsy is not known. However, various observational studies have identified the predictors of refractory epilepsy by clinical, imaging, and electrophysiological features. Clinical predictors of refractory epilepsy in symptomatic epilepsies include early age of onset of epilepsy, developmental delay, febrile seizures during childhood, status epilepticus at the onset, and presence of multiple seizures prior to treatment, multiple seizures after initial treatment, and focal neurological deficits. The best predictor of pharmacoresistance is failure of the first antiseizure drug, due to efficacy and not intolerance. Imaging predictors are presence of mesial temporal sclerosis, focal cortical dysplasia, and developmental tumors. Electrophysiological predictors include abnormal electroencephalography (EEG) in the form of frequent interictal epileptiform discharges. Given the failure of one appropriate drug trial, only 11% of patients eventually become seizure free, while only 3% become seizure free after failure of two appropriate antiseizure drug trials.

CONSEQUENCES OF REFRACTORY EPILEPSY

Drug-resistant epilepsy affects people living with epilepsy in multiple domains. Cost of medication, travel to meet expert doctors, repeated admissions, and expensive presurgical evaluation investigations lead to economical burden to patients and the family as well as to the nation. Psychological and social consequences of recurrent seizures and sometimes progressive deficits lead to irreversible disability. Recurrent seizures that interfere with school, work, and interpersonal relationships, during adolescence and early adulthood, prevent the acquisition of vocational and social skills necessary to live independently.

In addition, refractory epilepsy leads to additional problems in women in the childbearing age. They will have endocrine disturbances (weight gain, menstrual disturbances, excessive hair growth, etc.) due to multiple AEDs and will not get married due to stigma as well as due to fertility issues and risk of teratogenicity during pregnancy. They sometimes face marital discordance, if the disease was not disclosed before marriage.[7]

MANAGEMENT

Management of drug resistance epilepsy can be simplified into two steps. The first step is confirming the diagnosis of DREs, which can be partially addressed by general physicians as well. The second step is presurgical evaluation, which requires expertise in the field of epilepsy.

Confirming the Diagnosis of DRE

When patients diagnosed with epilepsy, and on treatment with single or multiple AEDs, report recurrence of seizures, one should follow a systematic approach, which includes:
- Whether patient is having epilepsy or not? Is it seizure or pseudoseizure or other nonepileptic condition or combination?

Approximately 10–30% of patients referred to tertiary centers as refractory epilepsy cases will not have epilepsy. They can have pseudoseizures or psychogenic nonepileptic seizures (PNES), syncopal attacks, paroxysmal kinesigenic dyskinesias, episodic ataxia, motor tics and paroxysmal symptoms of stroke, and demyelinating disorders. Most of these can be differentiated by careful history and reviewing the mobile video clips, if available.

Some important points that help to differentiate PNES from true seizure include gradual onset, on-off phenomenon in the semiology, prolonged attacks (>5 minutes to hours), eyes closed state, side-to-side head movements, bizarre limb movements, occurring only in the awake state and in presence of relatives, absence of injuries and incontinence, adolescent age of onset, variable and sudden increase in frequency, and associated psychosocial stressors. However, one should be cautious about making the diagnosis of PNES as around 10–20% of patients of true epilepsy can have pseudoseizures. In addition, some frontal lobe seizure semiology may appear like nonepileptic attacks. Hence, it is always advisable to follow-up the patients in addition to referral to a psychiatrist. These patients should be evaluated by a psychiatrist for associated comorbidities such as anxiety, depression, conversion, post-traumatic stress disorders, and personality disorders. Cognitive behavioral therapy and sertraline are effective in treatment of PNES.

Syncopal attacks are often wrongly diagnosed as seizures. These can be differentiated by history of attacks occurring in the standing position, brief duration of loss of consciousness preceded by lightheadedness, lack of postictal confusion, or headache. Vasovagal syncope is seen in children and adolescents where routine cardiac evaluations like ECG and echocardiography will be normal. Often head-up tilt table test with nitroglycerine challenge test is positive in these patients and can be used, if required.
- *Drug compliance*: Drug compliance is one of the important aspects with special challenges in our country with poor literacy and socioeconomic state of patients. Other causes of drug incompliance are poverty, lack of

availability of AEDs in remote areas, social stigma, and sometimes frustration, denial, and depression in patients for having to take medication for longer duration. All these issues need to be addressed patiently to ensure drug compliance.

- *Review of choice of drug and rational polytherapy*: When a patient is not responding to medication, after verifying the diagnosis and compliance, one should look for the appropriateness of the choice of the drug. The common mistake seen in most occasions is treating idiopathic generalized epilepsy with sodium channel blockers like phenytoin, carbamazepine, and oxcarbamazepine. Hence, one should verify the syndromic diagnosis of the patient. If it is idiopathic generalized epilepsy, consider valproate (avoid in females of childbearing age), levetiracetam, or lamotrigine as initial monotherapy (Table 1). If it is not controlled, a combination of these drugs can be tried. In case of symptomatic epilepsies, there are no evidence-based guidelines on rational polytherapy. As per expert consensus, one should consider multiple factors while choosing the combination, such as (1) choose the drugs with different mechanism of action, (2) avoid two enzyme-inducing drugs, (3) avoid drugs with synergistic adverse affects, and (4) select drugs with synergistic mechanism of action to control epilepsy. Among the various combinations, only the combination of sodium valproate and lamotrigine has some evidence as synergistic and has better seizure control.[8]
- *Dose is adequate or not?*
  Many times, inadequate dosing is the cause for uncontrolled epilepsy. Patients should not be given multiple drugs with inadequate cocktail dosing. Body weight of the patient should be checked and dosages should be optimized before considering therapy resistance (Table 2).

Table 1: Choice of antiepileptic drugs.		
Syndrome	Initial drug of choice	Second line
Idiopathic generalized epilepsy	Sodium valproate (avoid in females of childbearing age)/levetiracetam/lamotrigine	Topiramate, zonisamide, and clobazam
Symptomatic or cryptogenic epilepsy	• Carbamazepine/phenytoin/phenobarbitone/sodium valproate (avoid in females of childbearing age) • Oxcarbamazepine/levetiracetam/lamotrigine/lacosamide	Topiramate, zonisamide, and clobazam

Table 2: Dosage guidelines for established antiepileptic drugs in adolescents and adults.

Drugs	Starting dosage	Standard maintenance dosage	Dosing intervals
Sodium valproate	500 mg	500–3,000 mg	BID
Levetiracetam	500 mg	1,000–3,000 mg	BID
Lamotrigine	25 mg	200–300 mg (with valproate—200 mg or 3 mg/kg)	BID
Carbamazepine	200 mg	800–1,200 mg	BID
Oxcarbamazepine	300 mg	1,050–1,800 mg	BID
Lacosamide	100 mg	200–300 mg	BID
Phenytoin	100 mg	200–300 mg	BID
Topiramate	25 mg	200–300 mg	BID
Zonisamide	25 mg	200–300 mg	BID
Clobazam	10 mg	10–40 mg	BID
Phenobarbitone	60 mg	60–240 mg	OD

(OD: once in a day; BID: two times in a day)

Presurgical Evaluation

Once the patient is refractory to the two medications without any other caveats as discussed above, the patient needs to be referred to a neurologist/epileptologist. These patients require presurgical evaluation. The aim of the presurgical evaluation is to identify the epileptogenic zone and the functional deficits expected after surgery. Patients undergo various investigations as part of presurgical evaluation:

Phase 1: Clinical history, scalp EEG, MRI brain, video EEG (VEEG), and neuropsychological assessment

Phase 2: Magnetoencephalography (MEG), positron emission tomography-computed tomography (PET-CT)/MRI, ictal single-photon emission computed tomography (SPECT), and functional MRI (fMRI)

Phase 3: Invasive VEEG—subdural and depth electrode placement, and stereo EEG.

After each phase of investigation, patient will be reassessed. The number of investigations required varies from patient-to-patient. After the noninvasive evaluation, if the MRI can identify any lesion, VEEG shows matching semiology and ictal onset in EEG, and if it is in the noneloquent region, the patient undergoes resective surgery. If the noninvasive evaluation shows mismatch between lesion, semiology, and/or ictal onset, patient requires phase 3 evaluation of invasive monitoring.

If the presurgical evaluation cannot give a proper hypothesis epileptogenic zone, the patient is not a candidate for curative surgery. Palliative surgeries can be considered to reduce the seizure burden, prevent falls, and improve quality of life in some special situations, which will be discussed in detail in Chapter 16 (Surgery for Epilepsy). Other treatment modalities (palliative) available for treating these patients with refractory epilepsy are vagal nerve stimulation (VNS), responsive nerve stimulation, and ketogenic diet (KD).

Vagal Nerve Stimulation

Vagal nerve stimulation is an implantable treatment device, which consists of a small battery-powered stimulator. A fine-wire electrode extends from

Flowchart 1: Management steps.

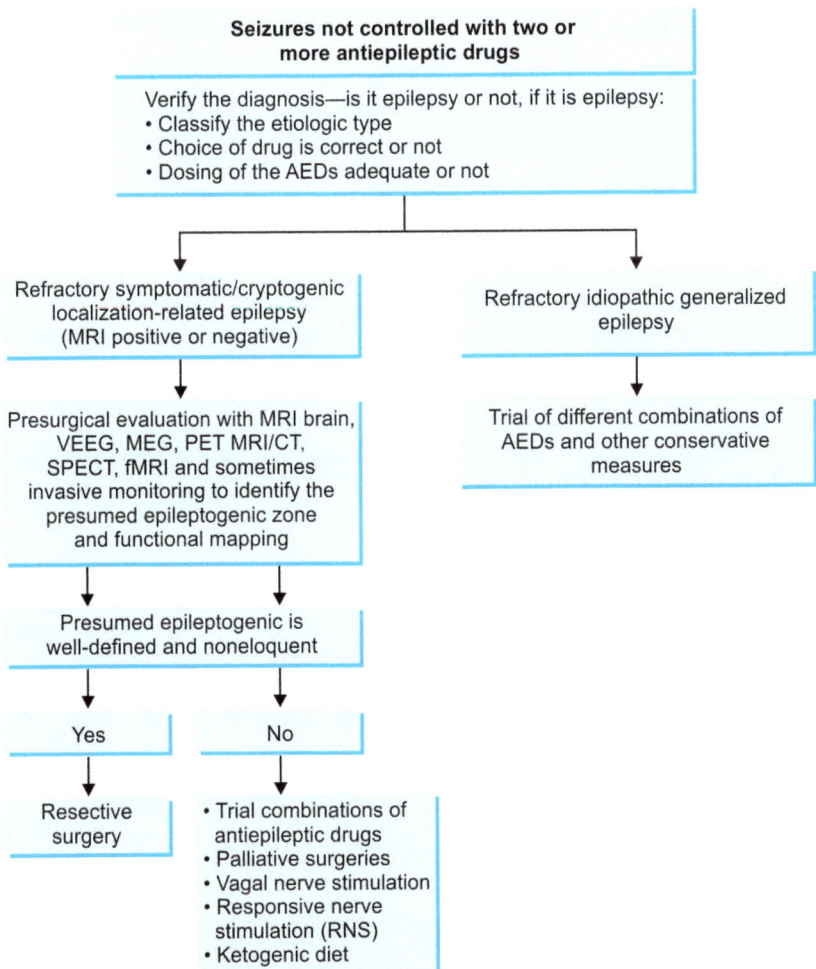

(VEEG: video electroencephalography; MEG: magnetoencephalography; PET: positron emission tomography; MRI: magnetic resonance imaging; CT: computed tomography; fMRI: functional MRI)

the device and is typically wrapped around the left cervical vagus. It is currently approved by FDA for therapeutic use in patients aged over 12 years with DRE. Approximately 40% of patients using VNS showed a 50% reduction in seizures after 2–3 years of treatment. The common side effects reported are dysphonia, hoarseness, and cough. These can be reduced by changing stimulus parameters.[9]

Ketogenic Diet

The KD, which is high in fat and low in carbohydrates, has shown a tendency to reduce seizure frequency. It is currently used mainly in children who continue to have seizures despite treatment with AEDs. Recently, there has been interest in less restrictive KDs including the modified Atkins diet (MAD) and the use of these diets extended to adults shows promising results for the use of KDs in epilepsy.[10]

The management steps are summarized in the Flowchart 1.

REFERENCES

1. Berg AT, Kelly MM. Defining intractability: comparisons among published definitions. Epilepsia. 2006;47(2):431-6.
2. Kwan P, Arzimanoglou A, Berg AT, et al. Definition of drug resistant epilepsy: consensus proposal by the ad hoc Task Force of the ILAE Commission on Therapeutic Strategies. Epilepsia. 2010;51(6):1069-77.
3. Sridharan R, Murthy BN. Prevalence and pattern of epilepsy in India. Epilepsia. 1999;40(5):631-6.
4. Kwan P, Sander JW. The natural history of epilepsy: an epidemiological view. J Neurol Neurosurg Psychiatry. 2004;75(10):1376-81.
5. Tripathi M, Padhy UP, Vibha D, et al. Predictors of refractory epilepsy in North India: a case-control study. Seizure. 2011;20(10):779-83.
6. French JA. Refractory epilepsy: clinical overview. Epilepsia. 2007;48(Suppl 1):3-7.
7. Kwan P, Brodie MJ. Early identification of refractory epilepsy. N Engl J Med. 2000;342(5):314-9.
8. Brodie MJ, Yuen AW. Lamotrigine substitution study: evidence for synergism with sodium valproate? 105 Study Group. Epilepsy Res. 1997;26(3):423-32.
9. Morris GL 3rd, Mueller WM. Long-term treatment with vagus nerve stimulation in patients with refractory epilepsy. The Vagus Nerve Stimulation Study Group E01-E05. Neurology. 1999;53(8):1731-5.
10. Martin K, Jackson CF, Levy RG, et al. Ketogenic diet and other dietary treatments for epilepsy. Cochrane Database Syst Rev. 2016;(2):CD001903.

16
Surgery for Epilepsy

Bhaskara Rao Malla

INTRODUCTION

In India, there are over one crore people with epilepsy (PWE), 20 lakh with drug-resistant epilepsy (DRE), and 5 lakh are potential candidates for epilepsy surgery (ES).[1,2] There is lot of progress in the understanding and management of epilepsy in the past two decades. If people with DRE can be identified early and referred to comprehensive epilepsy care centers (CECC), there will be substantial decrease in the overall burden of epilepsy.[3] Unfortunately for a number of reasons, PWE continue to suffer from the disease burden and are not benefitted by the recent advances. All people with epilepsy deserve proper diagnosis, medical management, and referral for surgery in suitable cases. With the establishment of a number of CECC in India, a sizable population of people with DRE can now undergo presurgical evaluation and surgical management.[4,5] In this chapter, basic concepts and strategies involved in ES will be presented.

GOAL OF SURGERY

The goal of surgery in epilepsy is to cure or control the disease. This goal is achieved in two ways: (1) Remove part of the brain where seizures start and (2) stop or reduce the way seizures propagate by disconnection or stimulation. Removal (resection) is possible, if we can identify structural (lesion) or functional (focus) abnormality of the brain and chances of cure or control of epilepsy is high. In disconnection and stimulation (neuromodulation), seizure burden will be reduced but cure or control is not possible in the majority of PWE.

SURGICALLY REMEDIABLE SYNDROMES

One of the recent advances in epilepsy management is understanding that some people with DRE do not respond to medicines, whereas surgery cures or controls their epilepsy.[6] People with mesial temporal sclerosis (MTS), focal cortical dysplasia, and low-grade tumors like to dysembryoplastic neuroepithelial tumors (DNET) and ganglioglioma belong to this category.

It is relatively easier to identify these people with simple noninvasive presurgical evaluation.

PRESURGICAL EVALUATION

In order to find out who will benefit and who will not following surgery, people with DRE have to undergo a standard presurgical evaluation. It aims to accomplish the following: (a) establish that the person is really having epilepsy and not pseudoseizures, (b) identify the underlying disease causing epilepsy (c) part of brain so identified, can be removed by establishing that vital functions (e.g. speech, vision, and movement) are lacking in the suspected region. The standard presurgical evaluation consists of careful analysis of the history, clinical features, magnetic resonance imaging (MRI) of the brain performed with epilepsy protocol, video electroencephalography (EEG) telemetry to record behavior and simultaneous EEG during seizures and neuropsychological assessment.

Neuroimaging

Magnetic resonance imaging has greatly helped in the evaluation of PWE who are being considered for surgery. It can detect almost 100% of structural lesions that are associated with epilepsy and can detect the MTS associated with mesial temporal lobe epilepsy (MTLE). High-resolution MRI can detect malformations of cortical development, neoplastic, gliotic, as well as vascular lesions.

Clinical Electrophysiology

Electroencephalography is the most important assessment in the study of epilepsy. It helps in identifying the epileptogenic focus. Magnetoencephalography (MEG) and stereo-EEG (SEEG) as well as high-frequency oscillations (HFO) are a few recent advances in the field.

Neuropsychological Assessment

Neuropsychological assessment is included as a parameter in the standard presurgical evaluation. It provides the best means to quantify the cognitive abilities and psychosocial status of a person. The pattern of cognitive strengths and weaknesses provides evidence for the area of cerebral dysfunction, also referred to as the functional deficit zone, which may overlap with the epileptogenic zone. In addition, neuropsychological evaluation also plays a unique role in assessing the potential risks pertaining to cognitive function after surgery.

SURGICAL PROCEDURES

Lesionectomy

Lesionectomy, in the case of epilepsy, is a surgical procedure that targets the structural lesion that is assumed to be the cause of epilepsy. With regard to isolated structural lesions, such as low-grade astrocytomas, DNET, or vascular malformations, excision is characterized by high-success rate. The approach for the surgery will often rely on the identification of the particular structural lesion preoperatively and intraoperatively. The surgical strategy adopted may include the following: (a) resection of the epileptogenic lesion, (b) extended lesionectomy, that is, resecting the lesion with margins, (c) resection of the epileptogenic zone and the lesion, and (d) resection of the epileptogenic zone without the resection of the lesion. In case of DNET, low-grade neoplasms such as ganglioglioma, vascular lesions like cavernoma, and arteriovenous malformation (AVM) and developmental lesions like focal cortical dysplasia (FCD), various surgical strategies for resection are adopted on the basis of the presurgical evaluation.

Anterior Temporal Resection

Mesial temporal sclerosis is the most prevalent cause of DRE. Anterior temporal resection (ATR) with amygdalohippocampectomy is the most frequently performed ES procedure. In ATR, 4–5 cm of lateral temporal neocortex, two-thirds of the anterior portion of the hippocampus, and two-thirds of the lateral portion of the amygdala with uncus and parahippocampal gyrus are resected. Surgery is tailored based on cortical vasculature, neuropsychological deficits, and cerebral dominance.

Extratemporal Resection

Extratemporal resection, in contrast to temporal lobe surgery, requires innovative surgical approaches and complex presurgical evaluation. Resection of small discrete epileptogenic lesions that are located in the extratemporal regions usually results in good outcome. ES involving the frontal lobe is prevalent in this category. Nonlesional extratemporal ES usually requires presurgical evaluation that is extensive and invasive, differing from one patient to the other corresponding to the noninvasive findings. Invasive EEG with strip, grid, and depth electrodes usually in combination as well as SEEG is essential to delineate the onset zone of the epileptogenic seizure.

Hemispherectomy and Hemispherotomy

Hemispherectomy or hemispherotomy is carried out to successfully treat hemispheric epilepsy that is medically incurable in the case of older children and adolescents providing impressive results with respect to seizure outcome and quality of life. According to the extension of anatomic abnormalities and the specific etiology, three different surgical procedures are carried out. These include anatomical hemispherectomy, modified functional hemispherectomy, as well as hemispherotomy.

Corpus Callosotomy

Corpus callosotomy is a surgical procedure performed to prevent propagation of epileptic activity from one hemisphere of the brain to the other. Disconnection syndrome is a known complication. However, with procedures performed before 10 years of age, disconnection syndrome is not reported and complications are a few. A lesion that can be resected should be completely excluded with thorough presurgical evaluation and workup.

Multiple Subpial Transections

The use of multiple subpial transections is particularly intended in conditions where the epileptogenic focus is located in the "unresectable" cortex, which refers to those regions in the cerebrum that subserve primary motor, speech, and sensory functions. The procedure is based on the evidence indicating that epileptogenic discharges need considerable horizontal or side-to-side interaction of neurons in the cortical regions and that the main functional properties of cortical neurons are dependent on the connections of the vertical columnar units.

Stereotactic Techniques

For temporal lobe epilepsy and generalized seizures, stereotactic techniques were practiced in India in 1960–70s. However, the establishment of image guidance has currently directed the use of these techniques for implantation of depth electrodes and SEEG for the localization of focus and to facilitate surgery.

Radiosurgery

In the past two decades, radiosurgery (RS) has been introduced for the management of DRE. RS is a method of treatment for people with DRE, wherein the focus of epilepsy is smaller in volume and can be radiologically well-defined. The classical conditions considered are hypothalamic hamartoma, arteriovenous malformations, and MTS. The outcome of RS has been described to be equivalent to what is observed with the surgical procedure. Nevertheless, the effects of RS on neurobiology in the long term have still not been identified.

Neurostimulation

Using electrical stimulation as a treatment for seizures, in patients who are not eligible for resective surgery, is a novel concept. The process of electrical stimulation is reversible. Additionally, if the stimulation fails to work, it is possible to discontinue and remove the implant. Its role is limited in India due to low cure rate and high cost.

Vagal Nerve Stimulation

The definite mechanism that is involved in the control of seizures by vagal nerve stimulation (VNS) remains unknown. It was perceived that continuously stimulating the vagus nerve using an electrical device that is implantable might lead to a widespread bilateral deactivation of the brain circuits that are considered to be involved in the generation of epileptic seizures. At present, this procedure is being recommended in certain cases of nonlocalized DRE. When compared with corpus callosotomy, VNS is more expensive, but is reversible.

Deep Brain Stimulation in Epilepsy

Deep brain stimulation (DBS) enhances seizure control in patients previously unsuitable for resective surgery. Stimulation of the subthalamic nucleus, centromedian, and the anterior nuclei of the thalamus, as well as amygdalohippocampal complex is carried out with partial seizure control.

Responsive Neurostimulation

Responsive neurostimulation (RNS) is performed by placing a small computer in the skull by connecting it to one or two brain regions that are epileptogenic, with the help of electrodes, permitting the identification of ictal onset followed by abortive neurostimulations. However, this procedure is not an alternative for resective surgery. RNS is indicated when resective surgery is not possible, for example, when two independent epileptogenic regions exist, like bilateral MTLE. Patients generally experience a reduction in seizure severity and frequency that is significant; however, they rarely end up being free from seizures. Results appear to improve over time.

Radiofrequency Thermocoagulation and Laser Intermittent Thermal Ablation Treatment

These techniques are indicated for lesions that are small and distinct such as hypothalamic hamartomas, MTS, and heterotopias. Applying laser intermittent thermal ablation treatment (LITT) for MTLE with MTS is an alternative to resective surgery. Post-LITT, when patients become seizure free, it might result in lesser neuropsychological deficits. In case their seizure episodes prevail, a second operation involving open resection can be carried out.

MR-guided Focused Ultrasound

Ablation with MR-guided focused ultrasound (MRgFUS) is a method that involves minimal invasion to generate focal lesions. In addition, MR thermography can be used to observe the extent of the lesion. The advancement in 1,000-array element transducers, improved focusing, and active scalp cooling has enhanced the interest in using transcranial MRgFUS for the treatment of epilepsy.

Pediatric Epilepsy Surgery

In pediatric patients, it is necessary to diagnose DRE at a much earlier stage, particularly in the case of children who present with catastrophic onset of epilepsy, epileptic encephalopathy, infantile spasms, and seizures that are frequent and disabling. In the case of children diagnosed with particular epilepsy syndromes such as Rasmussen's encephalitis, hemispheric syndrome, Sturge-Weber syndrome, and hypothalamic hamartoma, children should be advised to get a presurgical evaluation without delay. If children are identified to be suitable, surgery should be proposed at the earliest. Children that present with disabling and drug-resistant seizures with Lennox-Gastaut syndrome can be treated with functional procedures including corpus callosotomy to control drop attacks.

Complications

Interventional procedures can never be performed without the risk of significant intellectual, psychiatric, and physical complications. The impact of these complications does not just affect the patient and the surgeon, but it spreads to the family, referring physician, neurologist, referring organization, and society itself. Whenever ES is suggested, one must carefully assess the risks involved and the benefits. The preservation of cognition takes high priority. Inevitably, cognitive deterioration is a risk that surgical procedures carry. Nonetheless, control of seizure and reduction in medication can result in improvement of cognition. The potential risks involved in ES in the present times are acceptably low with morbidity less than 5% and mortality accounting for less than 0.5%. Complications during the surgery can include intracranial hemorrhage, cerebral infarction, intracranial infection, and direct cerebral or cranial nerve injury, possibly leading to temporary or permanent neurologic deficits. With respect to the patient's age and the surgery type, rates of mortality and morbidity differ; higher risks are associated with children in comparison with adults in corpus callosotomy and hemispherectomy, when compared with resections in the extratemporal regions and anterior temporal lobectomy.

CONTRAINDICATIONS

Primary generalized seizures, underlying metabolic or degenerative disorders or medical disorders that supervene and psychogenic seizures are contraindications to ES. Relative contraindications to ES include interictal psychosis, medication noncompliance, severely dysfunctional family dynamics, and severe mental subnormality.

OUTCOMES

Two randomized trials of surgery for MTLE with MTS reported 64% and 85% seizure freedom, respectively.[7] In frontal lobe resections, 1-year seizure remission rate of approximately 45% (range: 52-61) and less durable long-term outcomes are reported. In parietal lobe resections, Engel I outcomes range between 45% and 78%, with the best being associated with a focal MRI lesion. Occipital resections had an average Engel I outcome of 65%. In functional hemispherectomy, 73% of patients showed seizure freedom. Meta-analyses have indicated a 59% seizure reduction after anterior compared to the 88% reduction observed after total corpus callosotomy. In stereotactic RS, seizure-free outcomes range from 0% to 86%, showing a mean Engel I outcome of 51%. HH laser ablation resulted in 86% seizure freedom at a mean follow-up of 9 months.[7]

CONCLUSION

India carries an enormous burden of epilepsy. Surgery can reduce the burden of DRE. Like the rest of the world, surgery is underutilized and overly delayed in India. In spite of increase in the number of centers performing ES in India, currently, only one in thousand deserving candidates is actually undergoing the surgery. There is no doubt that we need more centers. But there should not be indiscriminate use of ES. Awareness and education of PWE as well as the healthcare professionals taking care of PWE are keys to the success. Recent publications from India highlighted the fact that early identification of people with DRE and referral to the CECC lead to not only cure or control of epilepsy but also improvement in the overall quality of life.[8-10] Collective effort of PWE, motivated healthcare professionals including physicians, pediatricians, neurologists, neurosurgeons along with the support of both governmental as well as nongovernmental organizations, is required in extending these benefits in medical and surgical management to large number of PWE in India.[11,12]

REFERENCES

1. Mani KS, Rangan G, Srinivas HV, et al. The Yelandur study: a community-based approach to epilepsy in rural South India—epidemiological aspects. Seizure. 1998;7(4):281-8.
2. Gourie-Devi M. Epidemiology of neurological disorders in India: review of background, prevalence and incidence of epilepsy, stroke, Parkinson's disease and tremors. Neurol India. 2014;62:588-98.
3. Berg AT, Langfitt JT, Cascino GD. The changing landscape of epilepsy surgery. Neurology. 2018;91(2):55-6.
4. Rao MB, Radhakrishnan K. Is epilepsy surgery possible in countries with limited resources? Epilepsia. 2000;41:S31-4.
5. Rathore C, Radhakrishnan K. Epidemiology of epilepsy surgery in India. Neurol India. 2017;65(Suppl 1):52-9.
6. Engel J. The current place of epilepsy surgery. Curn Opin Neurol. 2018;31(2):192-7.
7. Vakharia VN, Duncan JS, Witt JA, et al. Getting the best outcomes from epilepsy surgery. Ann Neurol. 2018;83:676-90.
8. Dwivedi R, Ramanujam B, Chandra PS, et al. Surgery for drug-resistant epilepsy in children. N Eng J Med. 2017;377(17):1639-47.
9. Dash GK, Rathore C, Jeyaraj MK, et al. Predictors of seizure outcome following resective surgery for drug-resistant epilepsy associated with focal gliosis. J Neurosurg. 2018;1:1-9.
10. Chaturvedi J, Rao MB, Arivazhagan A, et al. Epilepsy surgery for focal cortical dysplasia: seizure and quality of life (QOLIE-89) outcomes. Neurol India. 2018;66(6):1655.
11. Rathore C, Rao MB, Radhakrishnan K. National epilepsy surgery program: realistic goals and pragmatic solutions. Neurol India. 2014;62:124-9.
12. Rao MB. Epilepsy in India: Bridging the treatment gap. Neurol India. 2018;66:1060-1.

17
Epilepsy and Counseling

Akshita Hariharan

Individuals with epilepsy and their family members face multiple challenges such as illness-related stigma, dealing with restrictions in day-to-day functioning, comorbid health conditions, and ability to function independently.

Epilepsy can have a negative impact on family and social relationships, work opportunities, academic performance, and overall quality of life.[1]

IMPACT OF DIAGNOSIS

When a diagnosis of epilepsy is made, the patient goes through a range of reactions such as shock, fear, anger, denial, and confusion. The unpredictability of seizures makes them feel as though they have no control over the illness.

They seek answers for questions like, *"What is epilepsy? Why did this happen to me? Can it be cured? Can I go about my life as usual? Can I live independently? What will happen to me in the future?"*

The immediate family members of the patient feel helpless and concerned. They tend to react with overprotectiveness, anxiety, and restrict the person's activities due to fear of injury or death.

STIGMA

Stigma is perpetuated by the lack of knowledge. In the Indian cultural context, epilepsy is attributed to lack of spiritual faith, possession by spirits, karma for wrong doings, or insanity.[2,3]

Illness-related stigma affects economic status, psychological well-being, social interactions, and overall health even greater than the effects of the illness itself.[4]

Stigma can interfere with timely access to healthcare, early diagnosis, adherence to treatment, and lifestyle recommendations.[5]

There are two types of stigma as defined by Scambler and Hopkins[6]—enacted stigma and felt stigma. Enacted stigma refers to the acts of discrimination by others on the grounds of perceived unacceptability and inferiority. The patients face discrimination at the workplace/school and have to deal with hostility, abuse, neglect, and isolation by the society and extended family members.

Felt stigma is fear of negative responses from others, which leads to feelings of difference and shame. Felt stigma affects the patients' ability to carry on day-to-day activities, participate in social interactions, and has an impact on their self-confidence.

Patients and caregivers avoid social interactions due to the fear of having seizures in public, which leads to feelings of isolation, depression, and low self-esteem.

COUNSELING

Counseling the patient and family members at the time of diagnosis helps in reducing the stigma, improving compliance to treatment, and quality of life.[1]

A collaborative relationship should be established with the patient and family members. The physician needs to clearly communicate information using simple language and short sentences. The counseling should be patient-centered taking into consideration the age, life stage, and literacy levels. The patient should be encouraged to take an active role in the treatment and learn self-management skills.

The physician can take a proactive approach to counsel the patient and family members on the following domains.

Incidence and Prevalence

- Educate the patient about the current statistics available on epilepsy to help them understand that it is a common neurological illness that affects individuals across age, socioeconomic status, and literacy levels.
- Approximately, 1 in 26 individuals will develop epilepsy at some point in their lives.[1] Epilepsy is a treatable condition in 75–80% of people with epilepsy.

Information about Epilepsy and Seizures

- Communicate to the patient that epilepsy is due to sudden bursts of electrical discharge in the brain.
- Detailed history taking helps to make an accurate diagnosis. Investigations such as EEG and brain scans are recommended to get additional information about the illness and possible underlying causes.
- Different types of seizures need to be explained with emphasis on the type and pattern of the individual's illness.
- *Self-management tip*: Encourage patient to maintain a seizure diary to record the date, time, duration, and description of seizure, along with comments on possible triggers and postictal effects. Brief them about

the importance of keeping track of seizures, as it will help in modifying the treatment plan, if necessary. It is beneficial to hand over the format of the diary to the patient at the time of diagnosis.

Medications

- Help the patient to understand that medications are prescribed according to age, gender, current health status, and type of epilepsy.
- Inform the patient that the initial goal of the treatment is to reduce frequency of seizures. The duration of the treatment will differ from person-to-person depending on their response to treatment.
- Take a proactive role in informing the patient about the possible side effects of the mediations and how to cope with them.
- Poor compliance to treatment has been observed due to fear about side effects, forgetting to take the medicines, or unavailability of the medicine.[7]
- Emphasize the importance of strictly following the medication regimen in order to have the optimal effect of treatment. Give information on what the patient should do in case of missed dosage.
- *Self-management tip*: Counsel the patient to keep reminders/alarms to take the medications at the same time everyday (8 am and 8 pm). Use a medicine box to keep track of the medicines. Suggest modifying lifestyle to make it easier to remember to take the medicine (adjust meal times, keep medicine close to dining table, and carry medicines while traveling).

Triggers/Aura

- Educate patient about usual triggers for seizures such as lack of sleep, substance use (alcohol or drug use), high stress levels, menstruation, and missed dosage of medication.
- *Self-management tip*: Advise patient to be aware of the triggers or aura, so that they can move to a safe location and reduce the chances of injuries. Identification of aura and triggers helps individuals feel more in control of the seizures.

Restrictions/Precautions

- Counsel the patient regarding the activities they should avoid while on treatment, such as driving, operating heavy machinery, swimming, adventure sports, etc.
- Brief them about activities that they can engage in such as low-risk physical activities (yoga, cycling, football, cricket, etc.), carrying on routine tasks, participating in social activities, going to work or school, etc.

First Aid

Caregivers and family members can feel helpless during a seizure, counsel them on Do's and Don'ts during a seizure, so that they can provide the support/care that the patient needs.

- *Do's*: Remove objects from the surrounding to prevent injury, loosen clothes around neck, remove spectacles, turn patient to a side, and wipe away saliva postseizure.
- *Don'ts*: Panicking, putting items in hand or mouth during seizure, restricting movements during seizure, and giving liquids until patient is fully conscious.

Comorbidities

Discuss full range of comorbid conditions associated with epilepsy including mental health, cognition, neurological problems, and somatic disorders.

Age and Life Stage-related Counseling

Counseling is effective when it is patient centered. The requirements and concerns of the patients will differ according to their age and life stages.

- *Children:* Managing seizures at school, common learning problems, behavioral issues, symptoms of attention deficit hyperactivity disorder (ADHD), safety, and participation in extracurricular activities.
- *Adolescents*: Puberty, sexuality, alcohol and drug use, career, and vocational concerns.
- *Adults*: Employment, driving, marriage, and pregnancy.
- *Seniors*: Comorbid health conditions, living independently, and injury prevention.

When to Refer a Patient to Mental Health Professional?

A physician should refer a patient to a mental health professional when it is observed that he/she has:

- Seizure-like events (nonepileptic seizures) without electrophysiological changes, which are usually longer in duration with bizarre manifestations in movements and can be attributed to psychological causes or stressors.
- Symptoms of psychosis, anxiety, anger/rage, depression, and suicidal ideation.
- Need for emotional support, difficulty in carrying on routine activities, mood changes, and difficulty in accepting diagnosis or coping with illness, and nonadherence to treatment.
- *Cognitive changes*: Difficulty in paying attention, memory issues, difficulty in multitasking, and planning or managing responsibilities.
- *Children*: Behavioral issues, symptoms of ADHD, academic decline, and delay in development.

ROLE OF A CLINICAL PSYCHOLOGIST

- *Use of screening tools*: Beck's Depression Inventory (BDI), Hospital Anxiety and Depression Scale (HADS), and Neurological Disorders Depression Inventory in Epilepsy (NDDI-E) can be used to identify mental health-related comorbidities. The quality of life in epilepsy (QOLIE-31) can be used to identify the impact of epilepsy in the patient's life.
- *Cognitive behavioral therapy (CBT)*: It helps the patient to understand the role of thoughts in dealing and coping with the illness, and empowering the patient to take an active role in treatment. CBT can also help in reducing frequency of nonepileptic seizures and improve psychosocial outcomes in patients.[8]
- *Relaxation therapies*: These help to improve sleep and cope effectively with stressors.
- *Behavioral therapies*: Focus is on goals with clear rewards and feedbacks to promote positive behaviors and manage behavioral issues.
- *Supportive therapy*: It addresses adjustment issues related to epilepsy and provides information on how to communicate information regarding seizures and management to extended family members, teachers, and employers.
- *Neuropsychological assessments*: These are to identify cognitive issues and work on remediation to help the patient function adequately at school and at work.

Counseling the patient and family members can be a challenge in routine practice. During the initial consultation, the patient may not understand all the information given about epilepsy. It is important to be open to questions and address the issues that patients bring up over the course of treatment.

Educating the patient and family members plays an important role in adapting to life with epilepsy, developing self-confidence, and becoming competent in self-management. Support and care of the doctor and family members can help the patient to maintain a positive attitude, adhere to medical treatment, and live a full and rewarding life.

REFERENCES

1. Institute of Medicine (US) Committee on the Public Health Dimensions of the Epilepsies. Epilepsy across the spectrum: promoting health and understanding. In: England MJ, Liverman CT, Schultz AM, et al. (Eds). Washington (DC): National Academies Press (US): 2012.
2. Radhakrishnan K, Pandian JD, Santhoshkumar T, et al. Prevalence, knowledge, attitude, and practice of epilepsy in Kerala, South India. Epilepsia. 2000;41(8):1027-35.
3. Sureka RK, Sureka R. Prevalence of epilepsy in rural Rajasthan—a door-to-door survey. J Assoc Physicians India. 2007;55:741-2.

4. Baker G. The psychosocial burden of epilepsy. Epilepsia. 2002;43(6):26-30.
5. Thomas S, Nair A. Confronting the stigma of epilepsy. Ann Indian Acad Neurol. 2011;14(3):158.
6. Scambler G, Hopkins A. Being epileptic: coming to terms with stigma. Sociol Health Illness. 1986;8(1):26-43.
7. Hovinga C, Asato M, Manjunath R, et al. Association of non-adherence to antiepileptic drugs and seizures, quality of life, and productivity: survey of patients with epilepsy and physicians. Epilepsy Behav. 2008;13(2):316-22.
8. Goldstein L, Chalder T, Chigwedere C, et al. Cognitive behavioral therapy for psychogenic nonepileptic seizures: a pilot RCT. Neurology. 2010;74(24);1986-94.

18
Prevention of Epilepsy

Chanda Kulkarni

INTRODUCTION

Epilepsy is an eminently treatable neurological disorder. This section is dedicated to highlight preventive interventions in the management of epilepsy.

"Prevention is better than Cure" is an oft-repeated message, which also applies to prevention of epilepsy.

The World Health Organization (WHO) has proposed three levels of prevention—primary prevention as the one that involves averting the occurrence of a disorder, usually by reducing or eliminating underlying causes and risk factors; secondary prevention involves early detection or intervention to arrest or minimize the development of the condition; and lastly, tertiary prevention, which mitigates existing disease and its consequences through appropriate treatment and rehabilitation.[1]

PRIMARY PREVENTION

The recent report of the Prevention Task Force of the International League against Epilepsy (ILAE)[2] has suggested four major etiologic categories of preventable epilepsies.

Antenatal and Postnatal Care

- Poor and inadequate nutrition during pregnancy and perinatal brain insults are reported to cause seizures among children. Therefore, planned pregnancy is encouraged. Public health interventions to address maternal and child health care are important to follow.
- Administration of 400 micrograms (mcg) of folic acid everyday is important to prevent major birth defects of the brain and spine (anencephaly and spina bifida). Fortified foods or diet rich in folate are suggested.
- Anorexia in newborns and low birth weight are risk factors involved in seizure disorders. Hence, proper antenatal, perinatal, and postnatal care is essential to reduce complications during pregnancy and childbirth to prevent injury and risk for neonatal seizures.

Traumatic Brain Injury

- Severe traumatic brain injury (TBI) and skull fracture due to road-traffic accidents or falls are known risk factors of post-traumatic epilepsy. Measures to prevent TBI-like use of seat belts, safety seats for small children, air bags, bicycle helmets, and motorcycle helmets are recommended.
- Safety interventions such as assistance by caretakers, use of safety bars, wheel chair, etc. are suggested to prevent falls in the elderly.

Central Nervous System Infections

It is important to follow the current guidelines from the Public Health Programs in India for vaccination and immunizations to prevent infectious disorders. Effective and timely treatment of encephalitis or meningitis and cerebral abscess are necessary to minimize the development of epilepsy.

Cysticercosis caused by parasitic infestation, by *Taenia solium*, is transmitted through uncooked pork and in vegetarians the infection spreads through uncooked food handled by infected persons. This can be prevented by following good hygiene and washing hands prior to food handling. Deworming of school students with albendazole may be considered. A study to determine etiology using neuroimaging and investigations such as cerebrospinal fluid examination showed neuroinfection, as the leading cause accounting for 34% of which neurocysticercosis (35%) was the most common, followed by meningitis (29%), and cerebral malaria (17%).[3]

Cerebrovascular Disease

Cerebrovascular disease (CVD) is one of the main causes of epilepsy in elderly (>60 years). Population-based studies show that stroke increases the risk of epileptic seizure. Risk factors for stroke, e.g. hypertension, diabetes, obesity, hyperlipidemia, smoking, should be addressed to prevent stroke and consequent epilepsy.[4]

SECONDARY PREVENTION

- Factors facilitating the occurrence of seizures to be identified to prevent seizures. In patients with photosensitive epilepsy, the precipitating factors such as exposure to flickering bright/colored lights and flickering TV screen should be avoided.[5]
- Occurrence of repeated episodes of febrile seizures in children is known to increase the incidence of epilepsy later in life. Hence, appropriate and prompt control of febrile seizures in children until the age of 5 years is encouraged. The temperature should be brought down immediately by tepid sponging, ice pack on head, and antipyretics to present febrile seizure.

- In patients with hot water epilepsy, one should avoid hot water head bath.
- Deprivation of sleep is identified as one of the risk factors responsible for increase in seizure frequency. Therefore, persons with epilepsy (PWE) are advised to follow regular sleep pattern with adequate sleep hours (6-8 hour).
- Seizure disorders are also often associated with chronic alcohol and substance abuse and are considered risk factor for worsening of existing seizure disorder. It is therefore important to discourage use of alcohol and other substance use in PWE.

REFERENCES

1. World Health Organization. (2017). Health promotion glossary. [online] Available from http://www.who.int/healthpromotion/about/HPR%20Glossary%201998.pdf. [Last accessed April, 2019].
2. Thurman DJ, Begley CE, Carpio A, et al. The primary prevention of epilepsy: A report of the Prevention Task Force of the International League Against Epilepsy. Critical Review and Invited Commentary. Epilepsia. 2018;59:905-14.
3. Prakash B, Arun BJ, Ashok VB, et al. New onset seizures—an etiological study. Int J Adv Med. 2017;4:1532-6.
4. Dhanuka AK, Misra UK, Kalita J. Seizures after stroke: a prospective clinical study. 2001;4(1):33-6.
5. Wolf P. The role of nonpharmaceutic conservative interventions in the treatment and secondary prevention of epilepsy. Epilepsia. 2002;43(Suppl 9):2-5.

19

Epilepsy and Law

Srinivas HV

Persons with epilepsy (PWE), even when totally seizure free with appropriate antiepileptic drugs, face multitude of societal restrictions and have several hurdles to lead a normal life. They are denied admission to schools/colleges, sports activities, and social activities such as picnics, excursions, etc. They also have major issues for marriage and employment.

In this context, to assist PWE, what does the Indian Law say?[1] The following are some of the issues addressed. Medical professionals, PWE, and their caregivers should be aware of their rights.

EPILEPSY AND MARRIAGE

In 1976, the Government of India amended the Hindu Marriage Act and Special Marriage Act, which mentions that a person subjected to recurrent attacks of insanity or epilepsy cannot have a legally valid marriage and such a marriage shall become void, resulting in divorce. Through the persistent efforts of the Indian Epilepsy Association, the law was amended in December, 1999 paving the way for a PWE to have a legally valid marriage and epilepsy is no more an illness to claim for divorce.

EPILEPSY AND DRIVING

At present, Form 1 (Application-cum-declaration of Physical Fitness) has to be filled while applying for a driving licence". If the applicant responds positively to the question "Do you suffer from epilepsy or from sudden attacks of loss of consciousness or giddiness from any cause?", in spite of medical recommendation, driving licence is denied. In other words, even if the person is seizure free with or without medication, the word "epilepsy" in the application form denies the person a driving licence for life.

The Indian Epilepsy Association has been in correspondence with the Ministry of Surface Transport and Ministry of Health to amend the Motor Vehicle Act and grant driving licence with certain provisions. In Western countries, a person with epilepsy obtains a driving licence when he is seizure free from 6 months to 2 years, even while on medication.

EPILEPSY AND EMPLOYMENT

Persons with epilepsy obviously cannot be employed in jobs where one's life will be in danger, if the person has a seizure, such as having to deal with open machinery, live electrical installations, working at heights, etc. However, the ground reality is that all varieties of jobs including a desk job and blue collared jobs are denied to a PWE because of the myths and stigma attached to epilepsy. In western countries, there is a law to protect the interest of persons with epilepsy—the "Antidiscriminatory Law" which ensures that if a person is otherwise qualified for the job, he/she should not be denied the job on the ground of epilepsy. In India, we do not have such a law. However, one can still approach the courts, on the basis of one's fundamental rights.

EPILEPSY AND DISABILITY

The main aim of educating the masses is because epilepsy is an eminently treatable condition in 70-80% of patients, and PWE are entirely normal between seizures and can lead a very normal life. However, in the remaining 20-30% patients seizures may not be fully controlled or they have associated neurological disabilities such as hemiplegia (due to head injury, stroke, etc.), mental retardation, etc. The Disability Act recognizes the associated neurological disability and not the disability due to frequent seizures.

Any discrimination in education, employment, sports, and leisure activities on the ground of epilepsy can be challenged under "fundamental rights", as we do not as yet have an antidiscriminatory law.

EPILEPSY AND INSURANCE

Many insurance companies have a clause that they do not cover chronic illnesses such as hypertension, diabetes, etc. However, these illnesses are covered after a gap of 2-3 years. One should ascertain this clause for epilepsy whenever one is applying for health insurance.

EPILEPSY AND INCOME TAX

At this point of time, epilepsy is not listed as a disease for the purpose of deduction in income tax (80 DD).

REFERENCE

1. Epilepsy and Law in India Published by Indian Epilepsy Association—18th International Epilepsy Congress Trust, 2017.

20 Epilepsy: Education and Employment

Rajendra P Joshi

Epilepsy affects not only the patient but also their family in many ways. Education and employment are two important socially and psychologically important aspects, which concern most persons with epilepsy.

Education is a major concern, especially in children with epilepsy. Many myths and misconceptions are present in the society about education and epilepsy. There is a pressing need for spreading scientific knowledge about this aspect in not only to the person with epilepsy (PWE) and their parents but also to the general public, teachers, and even healthcare professionals.

Except children with other comorbidities like mental retardation or learning disabilities, most of the PWE are able to attend regular schools and their scholastic performance is found to be adequate.

The academic performance of a PWE may be affected because of modifiable factors such as depression, drowsiness secondary to antiepileptic drugs (AEDs), parental anxiety resulting in social restrictions, etc. Counseling, changing the formulation to slow release, or changing the AED helps to resolve the issue in many cases.

In a PWE, associated conditions like cognitive function and attention deficits can create issues at school and a poor academic performance. The resulting poor performance may be falsely blamed on epilepsy. A detailed neurological evaluation will identify the diagnosis.

Medical factors affecting scholastic performance are poor control of seizures, structural brain damage, multiple AEDs, higher dose of AEDs, and an early onset of seizures. Fortunately, these factors affect only a minority of the PWE.

In any PWE, the main treatment modality is AEDs. The present AEDs seem to have lesser adverse effects compared to older medicines and achieve good control with monotherapy in more than 70% of PWEs. The good seizure control itself improves self-esteem in the children and allow them to perform optimally.

Other factors such as decreased parental expectations, misconceptions about epilepsy leading to low self-esteem, and repeated absence from school are also important. Healthcare professionals at all levels need to specifically look at these factors and guide the family. Periodic psychosocial assessment, counseling, and support must be provided to improve the psychosocial adjustment in children with epilepsy.[1]

Please note that any recent onset of educational problems, PWE requires immediate and aggressive evaluation and management.[2] In such cases, a detailed history from the parents and teachers to clearly identify the problem is essential. Clinical examination is repeated to look for deficits and AED adverse effects. Monitoring of the antiepileptic drug levels in the serum, imaging, and electroencephalogram may be needed. Psychosocial evaluation to identify problems at home and in school is important.

Establishing good communication channels between the school, family, and the doctor goes a long way to help the child to achieve his/her potential. In addition to seizure control, sensitive monitoring to detect difficulties early and prompt remedial action is important. The parents and teachers should be encouraged to allow child to participate in leisure activities, which are safe and avoid unnecessary restrictions. The support for a child with epilepsy needs to change according to changing needs. A caring and knowledgeable doctor can make a huge difference in the life of a child with epilepsy.

Employment is another major concern in a PWE. While financial returns of getting a job are in itself a major and vital need for many people, the other aspects of employment are also important. A person with stable job will have an identity in the society and will have a structured lifestyle. His/her self-esteem will also improve. However, many studies have found that across the globe, a PWE finds it difficult to get employment and many a times settles for a lesser job than he deserves. It has been found that depression is less common in PWE with employment compared to unemployed PWEs.

A PWE can do most of the jobs and we have examples of great achievers in different fields to prove this. However, PWE should avoid jobs wherein a seizure can put either the PWE or others at risk of injury. Therefore, those having epilepsy are usually declared unfit for jobs of professional drivers of motor vehicles, construction workers working at heights, or factory work involving working near open moving machinery and certain categories of jobs in the defense services.

Even though a PWE has many options of gainful employment, there are many studies, which show that due to wrong beliefs or ignorance, they are denied many opportunities.

Many employers are reluctant to employ a PWE even though their seizures are under good control. In a study from Kerala, India, compared general population, the percentage of unemployment was significantly higher in the PWE.

In another study published in 2011, the main factors associated with unemployment in a PWE were poorly controlled epilepsy, recent seizure, lower educational status, and multiple AEDs.[3]

The effect of epilepsy on employment is widespread throughout the world. In another study published in Epilepsia in 2005, the unemployment rate for Korean PWE was as high as 31%. This unemployment rate was five times compared to general population. The quality of life of unemployed PWE was significantly lower than the employed PWE in this study. The employability of PWE was significantly affected by certain factors—the frequency and severity of seizures; age at onset; interseizure psychosocial disabilities including self-esteem, personality, and problem-solving style; and social discrimination. The study also states that actual discriminatory practices in the employment of the PWE were prevalent in Korea.[4]

To improve employment of PWE, only seizure control is not sufficient. In addition to seizure control, doctors should educate the PWE about employment and address their concerns to the extent practically possible. All factors affecting this issue need to be addressed including false beliefs in the society.

The whole society in general and employers in particular need to be sensitized.

Follow-up of a PWE should also include counseling and rehabilitation aspects. In specific cases, tailor made vocational training taking into consideration the medical aspects can make a huge difference.

The results of good counseling and rehabilitation efforts are noteworthy. In a study from the United States, nearly 43% of PWEs could achieve successful employment after vocational training. Healthcare providers should also become familiar with the vocational rehabilitation services available in their community.[5]

To conclude, education and employment are very important aspects of care of a person with epilepsy. The remedial solutions require proactive approach from the medical professionals beyond just seizure control. Healthcare professionals should use every opportunity to spread scientific knowledge about these social aspects of epilepsy.

REFERENCES

1. Singh H, Aneja S, Unni KE, et al. A study of educational underachievement in Indian children with epilepsy. Brain Dev. 2012;34(6):504-10.
2. Vinayan KP. Epilepsy, antiepileptic drugs and educational problems. Indian Pediatr. 2006;43(9):786-94.
3. Marinas A, Elices E, Gil-Nagel A, et al. Socio-occupational and employment profile of patients with epilepsy. Epilepsy Behav. 2011;21(3):223-7.
4. Lee SA. What we confront with employment of people with epilepsy in Korea. Epilepsia. 2005;46(Suppl 1):57-8.
5. Sung C, Muller V, Jones JE, et al. Vocational rehabilitation service patterns and employment outcomes of people with epilepsy. Epilepsy Res. 2014;108(8):1469-79.

21 Role of Yoga, Exercise, and Leisure Activities in Patients with Epilepsy

Inbaraj G, Sathyaprabha TN

INTRODUCTION

Epilepsy is identified as one of the most prevalent neurological diseases affecting over 1.5–2% of the population worldwide, with greater prevalence in the developing countries. It is a condition, which is defined as a susceptible state to develop recurrent seizures unprovoked by any known proximate insult. About 6 million individuals in India suffer from epilepsy. There is an assortment of medications available to enable individuals to control seizures. The objective of any treatment is to control the seizures, decrease the seizure frequency, the duration of seizures, and also to improve the overall quality of life (QoL). About 25–40% of individuals treated even with multiple antiepileptic drugs (AEDs) have uncontrolled seizures. They also encounter detrimental impact from medications, suffer from stigmatization, sudden unexplained death in epilepsy (SUDEP), and have a larger degree of psychiatric manifestations in contrast to humans with different illnesses.[1]

In India, a considerable number of epilepsy patients look for alternative therapies due to gaps in the delivery of modern healthcare to rural and some urban areas, socioeconomic challenges, poor social supportive network, difficulties in drug availability, compliance, and lack of awareness. In addition, a few patients prefer to opt for alternate therapy despite allopathic care being available. The benefit from complementary and alternative medicine (CAM) has reached a majority of patients in the recent decade, and studies have shown that up to 44% of patients are utilizing a certain type of CAM treatments including yoga and physical exercise.[2]

EPILEPSY AND YOGA

Yoga is an ancient traditional system of Indian medicine, known to mitigate stress and induce relaxation. It is known to bestow good physical, mental, and spiritual health with proven beneficial effects in epilepsy management. Practicing yoga is reported to reduce perceived seizure to a certain extent and also affects brain wave activity and arousal levels.[1] A recent study stated that 33.7% of the epilepsy patients found yoga to be beneficial in controlling seizures and a majority of them desired to practice yoga. It has been found that individuals who practiced yoga had a significant reduction in seizure recurrence and also dosage requirements of AED including their side effects.[3] We, at National Institute of Mental Health and Neurosciences (NIMHANS), have shown that autonomic dysfunction may additionally be a key factor causing SUDEP and hence enhancement in autonomic functions could be useful in lowering SUDEP risk. A multi-week (day-by-day for 10 weeks) practice of yoga has been shown to create a significant decline in seizure frequency scores and also better performance in autonomic function tests by enhancing parasympathetic activity. This signifies the importance of yoga as an adjuvant treatment in the management of autonomic dysfunction in patients with epilepsy.[4] Meditation stimulates the vagus nerve and decreases seizure frequency by 28–38% by modulating the limbic system and autonomic nervous system activity via hypothalamus. The conditioning of these regions by the practice of meditation is pronounced to assist the maintenance of normal homeostasis. Hence, stress reduction may play a pivotal role in clinical improvement and electroencephalogram (EEG) changes in these patients.[1]

Practicing Sahaja yoga provides persuading evidence of stress reduction by inducing elaborate changes in blood lactate levels, galvanic skin resistance, and urinary vanillylmandelic acid levels. A 62% and 82% reduction of seizure frequency was reported following the practice of Sahaja yoga at 3 months and 6 months duration, respectively. In the same study, the authors showed that power spectral analysis of the EEG demonstrated a shift in frequency from 0 to 8 Hz towards 8 to 20 Hz, indicating the impact of Sahaja yoga on EEG changes. They also provided evidence for improvement in visual contrast sensitivity using EEG and the Na-Pa [Na—the first prominent negative peak of mid latency responses (MLR); Pa—positive peak following Na] amplitude of MLR in primary idiopathic epilepsy.[5] Regular meditation is known to reduce seizure frequency and duration in drug-resistant epilepsy. Prolonged meditation also increases the background EEG frequency and reduces the mean spectral intensity (MSI) of the 0.7–7.7 Hz segment. This is accompanied by an increase in MSI of the 8–12 Hz segment. These results indicate a substantial improvement in the clinical-electrographic picture of drug-resistant epilepsy patients due to regular meditation practices. Therefore, yoga can be considered as a cost-effective method that improves the QoL in refractory epilepsy patients with minimal/no adverse effects.[1]

EPILEPSY AND EXERCISE

In 1968, The American Medical Association (AMA) recommended limitation of physical activities in people with epilepsy (PWE) due to the dread of seizure initiation or physical injury. Hence, PWE is restricted from participating in any physical activity and sports. Regardless of an expanding awareness and steps to restore participation of PWE, the social stigma remains till date and makes these patients less dynamic than normal individuals. Due to this nonparticipation, a decrease in aerobic endurance and self-esteem and an increase in body mass index, anxiety, and depression levels are common in epilepsy patients. Retrospective and prospective studies disprove the speculation that strenuous physical activities are injurious. This is gradually supplanted by the realization that being physically active is actually valuable in PWE. Despite the fact that there are rare instances of seizure occurring during/after physical activity, studies have clearly shown the vice-versa. In addition, it also uplifts one's cardiorespiratory and psychological prosperity. Sports, in general, are considered safe for PWE, provided special attention is given with close monitoring of medications. Physically exerting games such as hockey and football may not provoke seizures as misunderstood earlier, and thus PWE should not be precluded from participation. Special attention must be considered in sports involving heights such as gymnastics, horseback riding, and rock climbing. However, there are certain sports, which are not recommended due to the risk of serious injury or death, if a seizure was to occur during the game.[6] These include hang gliding, free climbing, scuba diving, etc. The benefits from physical exercise include improvements in both physical and mental health. An additional effect in seizure reduction can be observed when PWE engage in social integration during sports and this activity also helps in alleviating the stress levels.

During physical exercise, stress at certain limits can activate hypothalamic corticotrophin-releasing hormone (CRH). CRH, in turn, stimulates deoxycorticosterone release from the adrenal gland. This, in turn, induces an increased release of allotetrahydrodeoxycorticosterone from the liver and brain, thereby activating certain regions having GABAA (type A γ-aminobutyric acid) receptors, and effectively decreasing seizure susceptibility.[7] However, in spite of all these beneficial effects having high levels of stress can activate the hypothalamic-pituitary-adrenal axis, which leads to inappropriate release of adrenal and neural steroids, that can probably increase seizure susceptibility, which is a caution. A decrease in epileptiform discharges during physical exercise is the most established fact in many studies and should be considered in rehabilitation of PWE. Gotze et al. hypothesized that physical activity caused acidosis, which decreases the irritability of the cerebral cortex and thus increases the seizure threshold. It also enhances alertness and focus in an individual, further contributing to an increment in seizure threshold.[8] There are no studies confirming any established link between postexercise fatigue and high-seizure frequency.[6]

EPILEPSY AND COGNITION

Adults and children suffering from long-term epilepsy are known to be cognitively dull compared to normal healthy population. About a half of

PWE experience and display cognitive impairment in one or more domains, including learning, memory, attention, and executive functioning, with memory impairment being the most common. These deficits are directly linked to epilepsy pathogenesis or recurrent seizures causing physiological neuronal damage. The usage of AED is an another additive factor. They also greatly contribute towards poor QoL, which keeps them away from engaging in daily activities. There is loss of employment opportunities and economic downgrading also. Cognitive impairment is considered to be a central element for developing endogenous depression. Depression in epilepsy influences 20–55% of people who are ineffectively controlled on AED and also 10–20% of people with well-controlled seizures. This demands a higher degree of concern in PWE.[9] Hence, regular practices of yoga and physical exercise can show improvement in cognition and thereby help in reducing the depth and duration of low mood resulting in alleviation of the physical QoL.[9,10]

CONCLUSION

Complementary and alternative medicine therapies have turned out to be progressively prominent in the previous two decades. A strong evidence suggests that a large proportion of PWE are now using these treatments. This implies that physical activity and sports are a basic way to maintain both physical and emotional well-being. So, patients having epilepsy should not be excluded from participation in sports in view of causing injury or inducing seizures. More harm may be caused by discouraging physical activity and thus preventing its major benefits. A vast number of patients could definitely be benefiting from these adjuvant therapies, especially in those with refractory seizures. A well-designed, large, prospective, randomized study on these aspects is lacking and this might be the reason for scarcity in the evidence supporting the above beneficial claims of sports and physical activities in PWE. Regardless of methodological drawbacks of the studies, yoga and physical exercise can be considered an adjuvant treatment option for patients suffering from epilepsy.

REFERENCES

1. Panebianco M, Sridharan K, Ramaratnam S. Yoga for epilepsy. Cochrane Database Syst Rev. 2015;(10):CD001524.
2. McElroy-Cox C. Alternative approaches to epilepsy treatment. Curr Neurol Neurosci Rep. 2009;9(4):313-8.
3. Naveen GH, Sinha S, Girish N, et al. Yoga and epilepsy: What do patients perceive? Indian J Psychiatry. 2013;55(Suppl 3):S390-3.
4. Sathyaprabha TN, Satishchandra P, Pradhan C, et al. Modulation of cardiac autonomic balance with adjuvant yoga therapy in patients with refractory epilepsy. Epilepsy Behav. 2008;12(2):245-52.

5. Panjwani U, Selvamurthy W, Singh SH, et al. Effect of Sahaja yoga meditation on auditory evoked potentials (AEP) and visual contrast sensitivity (VCS) in epileptics. Appl Psychophysiol Biofeedback. 2000;25(1):1-12.
6. Pimentel J, Tojal R, Morgado J. Epilepsy and physical exercise. Seizure. 2015;25:87-94.
7. Arida RM, Scorza FA, Terra VC, et al. Physical exercise in epilepsy: What kind of stressor is it? Epilepsy Behav. 2009;16(3):381-7.
8. Gotze W, Kubicki S, Munter M, et al. Effect of physical exercise on seizure threshold. Dis Nerv Syst. 1967;28:664-7.
9. Allendorfer JB, Arida RM. Role of physical activity and exercise in alleviating cognitive impairment in people with epilepsy. Clin Ther. 2018;40(1):26-34.
10. Gothe NP, McAuley E. Yoga and cognition: a meta-analysis of chronic and acute effects. Psychosom Med. 2015;77(7):784-97.

22

Diet, Television, and Computer

Damodar Rao HK

There are many myths and misconceptions about diet, television viewing, and working with computers in persons with epilepsy (PWE). There is a need to clarify the above points not only to PWE but also their family members and caregivers. This will go a long way in spreading scientifically correct information in the society and also prevent unintentional wrong practices by the PWE.

It is observed that depending on regional and cultural practices, many PWE are put under diet restrictions, e.g. restrict fruits such as banana, spicy food, nonvegetarian food, etc. This may be because other conditions such as hypertension, diabetes, cardiovascular diseases have food restrictions. However, in epilepsy, there is no restriction as far as diet is concerned. The PWE can eat regular food like any other normal person. What is important is they should be counseled about the need for regular food timings and must avoid prolonged fasting.

Nowadays, television has become universally accessible and is part of social life. The main issue as far as PWE are concerned is that television viewing may cut short the regular sleeping hours. This is seen especially when there are international sports events. Hence, PWE and their caregivers must be counseled about the importance of regular sleep timings, as in some types of epilepsy, sleep deprivation may trigger an attack.

In some rare cases with photosensitive epilepsy, television viewing per se may trigger a seizure because of the flashing or repetitive patterns.[1] In such cases, PWE may be asked to take precautions such as watching television in a well-lit room with a lamp close to the television and watching from a distance of at least 8 feet. Prolonged viewing should be avoided.

Computer usage is rapidly increasing at all levels from students to working professionals. There are many doubts in the minds of PWE and caregivers about computer usage. There is no restriction on the usage of computers by the PWE. However, as described above, those with photosensitive epilepsy should avoid flashing or repetitive patterns on the computer when playing video games or watching movies on computers. In addition, the importance of regular sleep timings should be stressed while using computers as many people tend to work on computers late into the night.

While there are many myths and misconceptions about these common factors in the society, there is no need for any major changes with respect to diet, TV, and computers in a PWE. Importance of regular food and sleep timings should be emphasized.

REFERENCE

1. Prasad M, Arora M, Abu-Arafeh I, et al. 3D movies and risk of seizures in patients with photosensitive epilepsy. Seizure. 2012;21(1):49-50.

23

Indian Epilepsy Association: A Brief History

Muralidharan KV

INTRODUCTION

Epilepsy is a common neurological disorder affecting people across the globe irrespective of caste or creed. The disease is known to mankind since several centuries and unfortunately the stigma and myths attached to epilepsy continue even today in spite of scientific advances. This has resulted in untold sufferings for persons with epilepsy (PWE) who are discriminated in all walks of life—be it education, sports, employment, marriage, driving, etc. Today epilepsy is treatable in 80–85% of the patients. However, 100% of the PWE and their families suffer from deep social stigma, which is also responsible for the large treatment gap, particularly in the developing countries. While in other conditions like hypertension and diabetes, it is enough if one educates the patient and may be an immediate relative, in case of epilepsy the entire society needs to be educated to prevent discrimination of PWE.

INTERNATIONAL SCENARIO

The International League Against Epilepsy (ILAE) was founded by physicians in 1909, but its original intent was clearly inclusive, as Article IV of its first constitution, which clearly stipulates that "any person who is interested, either scientifically or practically in the work of the league can become a member of the league." Thus, nonmedical members could also become members of the international league through membership of the national organizations. The creation of a sister international association to represent PWE and their families and carers had been suggested by leading members of ILAE over the years. Perhaps, the most prominent of these was by the great American epileptologist, William G Lennox in 1939. However, it was only in 1961 that the International Bureau for Epilepsy (IBE) came into existence in Rome and the emblem—a candle—was also established at that time. Dr George Burden from the British Epilepsy Association became the first Secretary General of IBE. In 1974, a Declaration of intent was adopted to merge IBE and ILAE. Epilepsy International was, thus, established. However both—lay members and professional chapter—were reluctant to merge. The Epilepsy International was dissolved in 1985 and IBE resumed its separate identity. The IBE is an organization of laypersons and professionals interested in social aspects of epilepsy. The IBE addresses social problems such as education, employment, insurance, driving license restrictions, and public awareness. The IBE currently has 132 members across 100 countries. The IBE and ILAE work in close liaison and Joint International Conferences are held every 4th year.

BIRTH OF INDIAN EPILEPSY ASSOCIATION

Even in the early years, stalwarts in Neurology like Dr Baldev Singh and Dr EP Bharucha realized that contribution of nonmedical persons would be invaluable and immense in dispelling the myths and misconceptions attached to the disorder. In the late 1960s, some members felt that there was a need for forming a separate body to address different issues related to epilepsy—both medical and nonmedical. Dr Anil Desai was designated as the secretary of Epilepsy section within NSI and during 1968-1969, he along with Dr Noshir H Wadia totally involved themselves in creating a new society, without altering the constitution of NSI. This society would have members independent of NSI and laypersons could join in any capacity. The new society was named as the Indian Epilepsy Association (IEA) and a new constitution was formed, which included the essential objectives and rules under the Society Registration Act XXI of 1860. Dr Baldev Singh, Dr B Ramamurthi, Dr TK Ghosh, Dr EP Bharucha, Dr AD Desai, Dr NH Wadia, Dr KV Mathai, Dr KS Mani, and Mrs Roshan H Dastur were the members of the first Governing Council (GC) who registered IEA on 21 March 1970, in Bombay, and started having regular meetings.

In the first meeting held on 27 January 1971, Dr Baldev Singh was appointed as chairman, Dr Eddie P Bharucha as the Secretary General, and Dr (Miss) FN Kohiyar as Treasurer. This meeting, to ensure effective work in all important cities, took the decision to form local branches/chapters with at least 15 members each. The movement had an enthusiastic welcome. The central office in Bombay had 35 members (including nine founder members), Bombay branch had eight, Madras 25, Delhi 31, and Bangalore 24 members. The annual membership fee at that time was ₹ 10. IEA got a financial boost with ₹ 10,000/- being contributed by the PC Bharucha, trust much to the appreciation of all members. The GC on 18 December 1973 authorized Dr Bharucha to work toward the affiliation of IEA to the international body IBE and in the GC meeting at Vellore on 19 December 1974, it was informed that IBE had accorded affiliation to IEA. The affiliation provided us with an opportunity to host the 18th International Congress, in New Delhi, much before our own first annual conference, which was held in December 1993 at Chennai. The conference was attended by over 1,200 delegates, which not only gave immense opportunity for IEA to interact with several international delegates, but also provided surplus funds, which was pooled into forming a Trust—"IEA-18th IEC Trust", which was registered in 1992.

The IEA was initially managed by stalwarts like Dr KS Mani and Dr Bharucha as secretaries and subsequently by Dr VS Saxena and Dr HV Srinivas.[1] Today, IEA has 27 chapters.

ACTIVITIES OF INDIAN EPILEPSY ASSOCIATION

The duty of the central chapter is to guide and coordinate the different programs by various chapters including national and international conferences and symposia. The GC meets twice a year—in the mid-year at the proposed forthcoming venue of annual IEA conference and during the conference.

The GC deliberates various issues and formulates guidelines for the chapters so that the entire association activities are conducted in a cohesive manner.

ANNUAL CONFERENCES

Until 1993, only annual general body meetings were held on the sidelines of the Annual conference of NSI. The first scientific meeting was held on 23 December 1993 in Chennai along with the annual conference of NSI, which continued till 2001. From 2002 onward, it was clubbed with Indian Academy of Neurology (IAN) and conference was held for 1.5 days—the 2nd day mainly consisting of programs for nonmedical people. This was overlapping with the Continuing Medical Education (CME) program of IAN. The conference was in the same venue or in a different venue in the same city. Once the Indian Epilepsy Society (IES), which is affiliated to the International body—ILAE—was formed in 1997, joint annual conferences were held from 1999 onward. Gradually, the number of delegates—both medical and nonmedical—increased and it was decided to hold standalone conference from 2009 onward. The first one was held in Tirupati in 2009.

One of the landmark achievements is the amendment of the Hindu Marriage Act. Epilepsy was associated with mental illness and the spouse was granted divorce automatically. The association through public interest litigation fought this archaic law and with the help of various likeminded people, the act was amended and epilepsy was delinked from mental illness.

INDIAN EPILEPSY ASSOCIATION: BANGALORE CHAPTER

The IEA Bangalore chapter was formed in 1971 along with the National Body under the stewardship of Dr KS Mani with four nonmedical members. At present, the chapter has over 400 members and is involved in various activities that help in disseminating information and knowledge to dispel myths and misconceptions associated with epilepsy.

- *Public awareness programs* through street plays where a professional group of artists travel to interior villages, once a month, select a crowded place like bus stand, weekly bazaar and enact a drama that dispels the misconceptions associated with epilepsy. At the end of the play, various questions by the public are answered by a qualified neurologist who accompanies the troupe. This activity has been going on for the past 10 years and has already covered more than 600 interior villages.
- *Free counseling center and legal cell for the patients*: This activity is now extended to 5 days a week from the earlier twice a week.
- *National Epilepsy Day* was conducted on the 17th of November every year where a program with various activities are conducted, such as road show, public debate, essay competition for school children, painting competition for the young patients, and other public awareness activities. *International Epilepsy Day* is being conducted world over on the second Monday of February every year and so the National Epilepsy Day is now celebrated as International Epilepsy Day.
- *A quarterly newsletter, which* publishes various activities of the association, is mailed to all the members, neurologists, neurosurgeons, public libraries, and all medical colleges of the state.
- *Awareness campaign for student*: Catch them young and they are our future—with this motto, various schools (9th and 10th standard students) and colleges (preuniversity students) were visited to create awareness through a medium of drama and talks. Pre- and postprogram tests were conducted and it is happy to note that the message—busting the myths about epilepsy is well-received.

REFERENCE

1. Srinivas HV. (2013). A Saga of Indian Epilepsy Association: 40 Years of Journey. [online] Available from http://www.epilepsyindia.org/Images/asagaofindianepilepsyassociation.pdf. [Last accessed from April, 2019].

Appendices

Appendix-I

DO'S AND DON'TS DURING SEIZURES

Convulsive seizures (fits) top on its own, generally in 1-2 minutes and the following are the guidelines to be followed during the seizures:

Do's	Don'ts
Keep calm	Do not insert spoon or any such articles in the mouth
Loosen the tight clothes around his/her neck, e.g. neck tie, tight collar, and remove the spectacles	Do not restrict convulsive movements as it may cause fractures
Prevent the patient from injuring himself/herself	Do not crowd around the patient
<ul><li>After the seizure stops, turn the patient to a side and wipe the froth away from his mouth</li><li>If the seizure lasts longer than 5 minutes or repeats without recovery, call an ambulance</li><li>Do all you can to minimize any embarrassment; if the person has been incontinent deal with this as sensitively as possible</li><li>Stay with the person giving reassurance until fully recovery</li></ul>	Do not give water or other liquid until he/she is fully recovered

Appendix-II

FAMOUS PERSONS WITH EPILEPSY

Socrates	Greek Philosopher
Fyodor Dostoyevsky	Russian Novelist
Joan of Arc	French Saint and National Heroine
Charles Dickens	English Novelist
Sir Isaac Newton	English Scientist and Mathematician
Napoleon Bonaparte	French Emperor
Alexander the Great	King of Macedonia
Julius Caesar	Roman General and Statesman
Vincent Van Gogh	Dutch Painter
Lewis Carroll	English Author and Mathematician
Alfred Lord Tennyson	English Poet
Leonardo Da Vinci	Famous Painter
Theodore Roosevelt	American President during the Second World War
Alfred Nobel	Swedish Chemist, Inventor, and Noble Prize Winner
Martin Luther	King Junior, American Baptist Minister
Pythagoras	Greek Mathematician and Philosopher
Jonty Rhodes	International Cricketer, South Africa
Gustave Flaubert	French Writer
Saint Paul	Apostle
Heracles	Greek Hero
Arch Duke Charles	Austrian Warlord
Pius IX	Pope
Ludwig II	Duke of Württemberg
Lord Byron	English Poet
Hermann von Helmholtz	German Physicist
Vladimir Ilyich Lenin	Russian Revolutionist
Margaux Hemingway	American Actress
Tony Coelho	Former United States Congress Man
Tony Greig	Cricketer—Australian

Contd...

Contd...

Florence Griffith Joyner	Athlete—USA
Marion Clignet	Franco-American Cyclist
Chanda Gunn	US Women National Ice Hockey Goal Keeper
Agatha Christie	English Novelist
Michelangelo	Italian Sculptor, Painter

Source: Germany Epilepsy Museum. epilepsycentre.org.au, epilepsytoronto.org, Wikipedia

Appendix-III

MYTHS AND FACTS ABOUT THE EPILEPSY

Myths	Facts
Epilepsy is a mental illness	No, it is a disease of the brain
Epilepsy is contagious, so one should not come in contact with a person with epilepsy	Epilepsy is not contagious
Epileptic attacks damage the brain	Certainly not, on the contrary, it is the damaged brain, which can cause epilepsy
People with epilepsy are below normal in their intelligence	Epilepsy does not affect intelligence or memory. If the attacks are frequent or the person is taking large doses of antiepileptic drugs, this may affect the memory temporarily
Epilepsy is hereditary and so one should not marry	Epilepsy is not a hereditary disease. The tendency to get epilepsy is passed on in about 3% only. Hence, epilepsy is no bar for marriage
Epilepsy is lifelong disorder	Not at all, in about 75% of people with epilepsy, the seizures are well-controlled and a majority of them can go off the drugs
Epilepsy is rare	Epilepsy affects almost 1% of population all over the world
Seizures can be stopped by giving a key in the hand or making a person smell onion	False. The attack stops on its own
During an attack to prevent swallowing of tongue, one has to insert a spoon in the mouth	There is no need to insert any object in the mouth. In fact, this may cause damage to the teeth or gums
Epilepsy occurs only in children	Though it is common in children, epilepsy can occur at any age. In fact, a second peak of incidence occurs between the ages of 50–70 years

Index

Page numbers followed by *b* refer to box, *f* refer to figure, *fc* refer to flowchart, and *t* refer to table

A

Acetazolamide 52
Acidosis 49
Alcohol withdrawal 56
Alopecia, transient 102
Alpha amino-3-hydroxy-5-methyl-4-isoxazolepropionic acid 96
Alzheimer's dementia 32
Alzheimer's disease 43
American Academy of Pediatrics 23, 51
American Epilepsy Society 90
Anemia 102
   aplastic 102
Anion gap acidosis 73
Anorexia 102
Anoxia, perinatal 27
Antashubba 1
Anterior temporal resection 131
Antibiotics 43
Antibody
   antinuclear 38
   autoimmune 31, 38
   paraneoplastic 38
Antidepressants 43
   specific serotonergic 61
Antidiscriminatory law 147
Antiepileptic drugs 5, 12, 22, 32, 48, 56, 60, 74, 78, 85, 99, 101*t*, 115, 122, 126*t*, 148, 151
   adverse effects of 102*t*
   choice of 99, 125*t*
   induced cardiac malformations 49
   pharmacodynamics of 41
   pharmacokinetics of 41
   role of 60
   selection 44
   teratogenic effects of 49
Antiepileptic medications 44, 88
Anti-gamma-aminobutyric acid 31
   receptor antibodies 31
Anti-leucine-rich glioma-inactivated 31, 96
Anti-N-methyl-D-aspartate 31
Antipyretic drugs 13
Anti-thyroid peroxidase 37
Anxiety disorders 26, 58, 60
Apasmara 1
Arrhythmias, cardiac 41
Aspirin 14
Astrocytoma 36
Ataxia 92, 102
Atkins diet, modified 128
Atresia, pulmonary 49
Atrial septal defect 49
Attacks
   severe recurrent 15
   shuddering 17
   transient ischemic 30, 41, 43
Attention-deficit hyperactivity disorder 26, 65
Autism-spectrum disorders 26
Autonomic function tests 30
Autosomal dominant 70
   disorder 11
   frontal lobe epilepsy 70
   juvenile myoclonic epilepsy 70
   nocturnal frontal lobe epilepsy 69
   partial epilepsy with auditory features 70

B

Bangalore Urban and Rural Neuroepidemiological Survey 42
Beck's depression inventory 141
Behavioral changes 102
Behavioral problems 111
Behavioral therapies 141
Benzodiazepines 105
   gamma-aminobutyric acid 60
   oral 88
   parenteral 89
   trial 95*f*
Biochemical tests 77
Bone marrow depression 102
Bradyarrhythmia 55
Brain 1, 73, 99
   damage
      risk of 15
      structural 56
   disorder of 30
   human 4
   injury, traumatic 36, 43, 144
   neurotransmitters 45
   presence of 8
   tumor 36, 90
Breath-holding spell 10, 17, 18
Brivaracetam 105
Broad-spectrum parenteral anticonvulsants effective against multiple seizure types 89
Brudzinski signs 10

C

Calcification 83
Calcium 8
Carbamazepine 5, 33, 44, 49, 60, 72, 100-103, 116, 125, 126
Cardiopulmonary resuscitative procedures 15
Carotid sinus syndrome 41
Catamenial epilepsy 52
Catastrophic seizure syndromes 28
Cavernous angiomas 32
Central nervous system 32, 34, 89
    infection 10, 144
        rule out 10
Centrotemporal spikes 80, 110
Cerebrovascular disease 144
Charaka Samhita 1
Chest
    infections 42
    X-ray of 43
Chills 10
Chromosomal microarray 75
Clinical psychologist, role of 141
Clobazam 33, 52, 92, 101, 102, 105, 125, 126
    oral 88
Clonazepam 92, 102
Cognitive behavioral therapy 61, 141
Commissure
    anterior 82
    posterior 82
Commitment therapy 61
Comprehensive epilepsy care centers 129
Computed tomography 126, 127
    scan 112
Computer 156
Confusion 92, 102
Consciousness 94f
    assessment of 10
Continuous therapy 13
    indications for 13
Contraception 51
Conventional antiepileptic drug therapy 23
Convulsions
    neonatal 27
    study of 2
Convulsive diseases, chronic 3
Corpus callosotomy 132
Cortical development, malformations of 24, 25
Corticotrophin-releasing hormone 153
Cough syncope 55
Craniofacial defects 49
Cysticercosis 89

D

De novo
    mutation 11
    psychosis after epilepsy surgery 63
Deep brain stimulation 133

Deep tendon reflex, assessment of 10
Dementias 43, 90
Deoxyribonucleic acid 71
Depression 58, 102
    cardiac 92
    respiratory 92
    screening for 60
    treatment strategies for 60
Depressive disorder 26
Diabetes 55
    gestational 49
Diazepam 13, 90
    oral 88
Diet 156
Diffusion-tensor imaging 83
Diffusion-weighted image 34
Diphtheria/tetanus/pertussis 8
Diplopia 102
Divalproate 60
Dizziness 102
Doose syndrome 68
Doshas 1
Down syndrome 90
Dravet syndrome 8, 10, 11, 26, 68, 72, 111
Drop attacks 18, 28
Drowsiness 92
Drug 56
    compliance 124
    resistant epilepsy 105, 122, 123, 129
        management of 123
    withdrawal
        after seizure freedom 115
        benefits of 116
        risks of 117
Duloxetine 61
Dysautonomia, primary 55
Dysembryoplastic neuroepithelial tumors 24, 129
Dyskinesia, paroxysmal 30
Dyslipidemia 26
Dysplasia 24
    focal cortical 32, 83, 131

E

Edema, perilesional 35f
Electrocardiogram 30, 43
Electroclinical syndromes 90
Electroconvulsive therapy 93
Electroencephalogram 3, 11, 18, 20, 22, 31, 42, 63, 107, 152
Electroencephalography 77, 85fc, 99, 112, 117, 123
    abnormalities 80t
    continuous 93
    role of 93
Electrolytes, serum 43
Electrophysiological procedures 80
Electrophysiology 77
    clinical 130

Elekta Neuromag® Triux
    Magnetoencephalography Machine 81*f*
Encephalitis 10, 55, 90, 111
    autoimmune 32, 37, 96
    viral 56
Encephalopathy 92
    autoimmune 31
    developmental 23
    epileptic 16, 23, 69, 72
    hepatic 56
    metabolic 56
    mitochondrial 70
    renal 56
    steroid-responsive 37
Enzyme
    inducibility 45
    induction 92
Ephedrine 32, 56
Epigenetics 71
Epilepsy 1-3, 6, 16-19, 26, 30, 36, 42, 46, 48, 54, 56, 56*t*, 58, 61, 64, 65, 67, 77, 77*t*, 83, 85, 99, 104, 107, 109, 133, 137, 138, 143, 148, 151, 158
    absence of 65, 80
    adult-onset 16, 34
    and cognition 153
    and counseling 137
    and disability 147
    and driving 146
    and employment 147
    and epilepsy syndromes 16
    and exercise 152
    and functional anatomy 4
    and income tax 147
    and insurance 147
    and law 146
    and marriage 146
    and psychiatric aspects 58
    and yoga 151
    anxiety disorders in 60
    benign 26
    childhood 16, 17, 21, 25, 26, 80
    classification 28, 107
    cryptogenic 125
    development of 14
    diagnosis of 41, 80, 107, 109, 112
    education and employment 148
    emergencies in 88
    epidemiology of 41
    etiology of 41
    famous persons with 164
    focal 109, 110
    frontal lobe 18, 65
    generalized 8, 25, 109, 110
    genetic 67
        basis of 67
        causes of 69, 73
        diagnosis of 67
    history of 1
    idiopathic 16, 31
    generalized 68, 80, 110, 122, 125
    in elderly 41
    investigation of 77, 112
    juvenile
        absence 90, 110, 122
        myoclonic 31, 32, 51, 64, 79, 80, 110, 116, 122
    management of 4, 52, 143
    medical treatment of 73, 99
    medically refractory 73, 105
    mesial temporal 33, 83, 130
    metabolic 111
    mitochondrial 72
    myoclonic 32, 70
    neurological disorders depression inventory for 60, 141
    new-onset 30-32, 38
        idiopathic generalized 100
        partial 100
    on pregnancy 48
    pediatric 25, 27, 28, 134
    pharmacokinetics of 73
    pharmacoresistant 27
    phenotypic characteristics of 16
    post-traumatic 36
    prevention of 143
    primary
        generalized 94*f*
        new-onset 31
    protocol magnetic resonance imaging 82*t*
    pyridoxine-dependent 72
    recent classification of 116
    refractory 105, 105*t*, 122, 123
    secondary new-onset 34
    self-limited 110
        occipital 110
    severe myoclonic 8
    short history of 1
    stigma of 54
    sudden unexplained death in 151
    surgery for 129
    symptomatic 16, 25, 125
        focal 24
    syndrome 18, 20, 20*t*, 21, 22, 67, 110, 110*t*
        febrile infection-related 10, 11, 90
        identification of 110
        self-limiting focal 21*t*
        specific 26
    temporal lobe 59, 64, 68, 80
    therapy resistance in 122
    treatment of 6, 41
    types of 80
    with complex inheritance 69
Epileptic syndrome 11, 31, 42, 80*t*
Epileptiform discharges, absence of 112
Epileptogenic lesions 83*t*
Erythrocyte sedimentation rate 34
Escitalopram 61

Eslicarbazepine 101
Ethosuximide 102
European Association of Epilepsy Centers 5
European Forum on Epilepsy Research 6
Everolimus 72
Exercise, role of 151
Extratemporal resection 131
Ezogabine 72

F

Falling disease 1
Fallot's tetralogy 49
Father of medicine 1
Fatigue 92, 102
    paresthesias 102
Febrile
    delirium 10
    episode 13
    myoclonus 10
    seizures 7-9, 14, 15, 23, 56
        development of 8
        first 12
        majority of 11
        plus 68, 70
            syndrome 8, 25
        treatment of 11
Felbamate 101, 102
Fenfluramine 72
Fetal
    heart rate 49
    hypoxia 49
Fever 10
    causes of 10
    infections 8
    low-grade 12
Fluid attenuated inversion recovery 34, 82
Fluoxetine 61
Folic acid 8
Fosphenytoin 12, 92
Functional magnetic resonance imaging 84*f*

G

Gabapentin 43, 100, 104
Gait problems 111
Galen's theory 2
Gamma-aminobutyric acid 8, 96
Ganglioglioma 24, 83
Gastroenteritis 8
Gastrointestinal
    irritation 102
    malformations 49
Gator1 complex 72
Genetic 8
    epilepsy 16, 31, 70, 71, 74*fc*, 118
        syndromes 70*t*
    etiology 19
    factors 8

generalized epilepsy 110
    testing 11
Genomic imprinting, disorder of 73
Ginkgo biloba 43
Glaucoma 102
Gliosis 111
Global Campaign Against Epilepsy 5
Glucose
    transporter deficiency 71, 72
        syndrome 27
Glucuronidation, hepatic 51
Glutamic acid decarboxylase 96
Granulomas 34
    cysticercal 32
    neurocysticercal 34*t*
    tuberculous 34*t*
Growth hormone deficiency 26
Gum hyperplasia 102

H

Hamartoma, hypothalamic 19, 25
Hans Berger 3
Hashimoto's encephalopathy 37
Head
    injury 56
    trauma 36
Headache 102
Hearing 73
    loss, sensorineural 69
Heart 73
    disease, structural 41
Hemiconvulsion-hemiplegia epilepsy 19
Hemiparesis, transient 9
Hemispherectomy 131
Hemispherotomy 131
Hemogram 43
Hemorrhage 49
    postpartum 49
Henri Jean Pascal Gastaut 4
Hepatic failure 102
Hepatotoxicity 13, 93, 102
Herpes
    encephalitis 32
    simplex 55
Hippocrates 2
Hirsutism 102
Histone modifications 71
Holter monitoring 30
Hospital Anxiety and Depression Scale 141
Human immunodeficiency virus 32, 36
Hydronephrosis 49
Hyperammonemia 13, 73, 92, 102
Hyperekplexia 17
Hyperglycemia 32, 41, 42
Hypernatremia 32, 41
Hyperphagia 64, 65
Hypersexuality 64
Hypertensive disorders 49

Hyperthermia 64
Hypnic jerks 41
Hypocalcemia 30, 32, 34, 41, 42, 44, 54, 56, 73
Hypohidrosis 102
Hypometabolism, severe 84*f*
Hyponatremia 32, 34, 41, 42, 56, 102
Hypospadias 49
Hypotension 92
    orthostatic 41
Hypothermia, therapeutic 93
Hypothyroidism 26, 42
Hypoxia, maternal 49
Hypsarrhythmia 80

I

Immunization 8
Immunoglobulin 37
Indian Academy of Neurology 160
Indian Epilepsy Association 6, 146, 158-160
    activities of 160
    birth of 159
Infantile spasm 18, 26, 69
Infections 34, 111
    extracranial 8
Infertility 48
Insomnia 102
Intensive care unit 96
Interictal epileptiform discharges 78
Intermittent therapy 13
    indications for 13
International 10-20 Montage System 79*f*
International Bureau for Epilepsy 158
International Classification of Epileptic
    Seizures and Epilepsies 5
International Epilepsy Day 161
International League Against Epilepsy 4, 18,
    67, 116, 158
    Classification of Seizure Types Basic
        Version 108*f*
    Classification of Seizures and Epilepsies 107
    Framework for Classification of
        Epilepsies 108*f*
International Neuropsychiatric Interview Plus 60
Intoxication 90
Intracranial infection, acute 7
Intrauterine
    device 51
    growth retardation 9
Iron 8

J

Japanese encephalitis 55
Jitteriness 17
John Hughlings Jackson 2

K

Kapha 1

Kernig's signs 10
Ketamine 93
Ketogenic diet 72, 93, 128
Kidney 73
Klüver-Bucy syndrome 64

L

Lacosamide 12, 33, 92, 105, 125, 126
Lactic acidosis 70
Lafora's disease 69, 85, 90
Lamotrigine 33, 43, 48, 72, 100-102, 125, 126
Landau-Kleffner syndrome 26
Language impairment 26
Laser intermittent thermal ablation treatment
    133
Learning disability 111
Lennox-Gastaut syndrome 3, 4, 26, 69, 80, 90,
    104
Lesionectomy 131
Lethargy 102
Leukopenia 102
Levetiracetam 12, 33, 43, 92, 100-102, 125, 126
Levodopa 43
Limbic encephalitis 23
Liver 73
    enzymes, elevated 92
    failure 42, 105
    function tests 43
Lorazepam 90, 95*f*
Lumbar puncture 11, 96
Lymphadenopathy 102

M

Magnetic resonance imaging 11, 77, 81, 83*t*,
    84*f*, 85*f*, 99, 112, 127, 130
Magnetoencephalography 126, 127, 130
Malaria 90
Malformations
    arteriovenous 32
    major congenital 49
Manganese 8
Marriage, low rates of 48
Masturbation 17, 64
Mean spectral intensity 152
Memantine 72
Memory disorders 65
Mendelian inheritance 69
Meningeal irritation, signs of 10
Meningioma 36
Meningitis 10
    bacterial 56
    cryptococcal 36
Menstrual irregularities 48
Mental
    disorders, statistical manual of 59
    retardation 27
    stress 48

Metabolism
    hepatic 45
    inborn error of 73
    several inborn errors of 23
Metastatic lesions 36
Methylation 71
Micturition syncope 55
Midazolam 88, 91, 93
Midline craniofacial anomalies 49
Migraine 17, 18
    complicated 30
Miscarriages 49
Mitochondrial
    disease 69
    inheritance 69, 70
    syndromes 85
Mood
    disorders 26
    symptoms 64
Morbus Divus 2
Morbus Sacer 2
Motor disabilities 111
Motor vehicle Act 146
Movement disorders 30, 111
Multifocal paraneoplastic disorders 23
Multiorgan involvement 34, 73
Multiple subpial transections 28, 132
Muscle 73
    biopsy 77
    oligodendrocyte glycoprotein 37
    tone and power, assessment of 10
Myoclonic disease, severe 69
Myoclonus 92
Myopathy sensory ataxia 70

N

Narcolepsy 41
National Epilepsy Day 161
National Institute of Mental Health and Neurosciences 152
Neonatal epilepsy, benign familial 69, 70
Neonatal intensive care unit 9
Nerve 73
Nervous system malformations 49
Neural tube defects 49
Neurocysticercosis 34, 35f
Neuroleptics 43
Neurological disorder, chronic 58
Neurological Society of India 6
Neuromyelitis optica 37
Neuronal ceroid lipofuscinosis 85
    adult-onset 32
Neurons, epileptic 4
Neuropsychiatric disorder, developmental 25
Neurostimulation 133
    responsive 133
Neurosyphilis 32, 36
Neurotuberculosis 34

Nimesulide 14
N-methyl-D-aspartate 23, 96
Nonepileptic attack 30
    disorder 54, 56, 56t
Nonmendelian inheritance 69
Norepinephrine-dopamine reuptake inhibitors 61

O

Obsessive compulsive disorder 65
Ocular hypertelorism 49
Oligodendroglioma 36
Orbitofrontal lesions 65
Osteomalacia 102
Otitis media 8
Oxcarbamazepine 125, 126
Oxcarbazepine 33, 100-102

P

Panayiotopoulos syndrome 21, 90
Pancreatitis 92
Panic attacks 55
Papilledema 10
Paracetamol oral 13, 15
Parenchymal hemorrhagic lesions 36
Paresthesias 92
Parkinson's disease 55
Paroxysmal torticollis, benign 17
Paroxysmal vertigo, benign 17
Patent ductus arteriosus 49
Pediatric neurologic disorders 16
Pentobarbital 93
Perampanel 105
Persons with epilepsy 1, 58, 115, 129, 145, 146, 148, 152, 156, 158
Phenobarbital 50, 101, 105
Phenobarbitone 12, 13, 92, 100, 102, 116, 125, 126
Phenylephrine 32, 56
Phenytoin 5, 44, 50, 92, 94f, 100-103, 116, 125, 126
    intravenous 12
Phosphorus metabolism 41
Pitta 1
Pleitropy 67
Pneumonia 8
Polycystic ovary syndrome 26
Polymicrogyria 24
Polypharmacy 45
Porphyria 105
Positron emission tomography 5, 77, 83, 84f, 126, 127
Premature birth 8
Presyncope 30
Prevention Task Force of International League Against Epilepsy 143
Primidone 49, 104

Propofol 93
Protein binding 45
Pseudocrisis 18
Pseudoseizures 124
Psychiatric
    comorbidities 26
    conditions 111
Psychic blindness 64
Psychogenic crises 17
Psychosis 26, 61-63, 102
    chronic interictal 63
    in persons with epilepsy 61
    interictal 65
    postictal 62
    prevalence of 61
Public Awareness Programs 161
Pyridoxine 27, 72, 93

Q

Quinidine 72
Quinolones 32, 56

R

Radiofrequency thermocoagulation 133
Radiosurgery 132
Randomized controlled trials 46
Rapamycin inhibitors, mammalian target of 72
Rapid eye movement 41
Rasmussen syndrome 19
Rectal preparation 12, 14
Regression, developmental 73
Renal agenesis 49
Renal failure 104
Renal function tests 43
Renal stones 102
Respiratory rate, monitor for 91
Restless legs syndrome 41
Retigabine 101
Ribonucleic acids 71
    noncoding 71
Rolandic epilepsy 80
Rolandic seizure 18

S

Sandifer syndrome 17, 18
Sclerosis
    hippocampal 19, 82, 111
    mesial temporal 24, 31-33, 95f, 129, 131
    multiple 37
    tuberous 72
Sedation 102
Seizures 3, 8-11, 17, 19, 48, 54, 55, 55t, 69, 88, 107, 138
    absence 11, 18
    acute 44
        repetitive 88

and epilepsy, first unprovoked 43
atonic 11
characteristics 10
cluster 88
complex
    febrile 9, 9t, 59
    partial 79f
convulsive 163
differential diagnoses of 41b
disorders 145
drug induced 34
duration of 10
during pregnancy, recurrence of 48
early-onset 36
epileptic 30, 115, 117
focal 18, 19, 31
frequency 52
generalized 16, 19, 109
hysterical 54
isolated 34, 88
migrating partial 72
myoclonic 11, 18
neonatal 73
nonepileptic psychogenic 41
occipital lobe 18
paradoxical worsening of 92
poststroke 34, 36
post-traumatic 34, 36
prolonged febrile 11
provoked 42, 56b
psychogenic 54
    nonepileptic 124
reduction 28
re-emergence of 49
sensory 41
simple febrile 9, 9t
temporal lobe 18
types 18, 20-22
    classification of 19b
    identification of 107
typical febrile 68
Selective serotonin-norepinephrine reuptake inhibitors 61
Selenium 8
Sertraline 61
Sexual maturation-related issues 26
Single-photon emission computed tomography 77, 83, 126
Skin 77
    rash 102
Sleep
    apnea 41
    benign epileptiform transients of 112
    deprivation of 145
    positive occipital sharp transients of 112
    myoclonus, venign 17, 18
    disorders 17, 18, 30, 41, 111
Sodium
    channel blocker 72
    valproate 5, 32, 49, 116, 125, 126

Somnolence 92
Spasm, march of 2
Spasmus nutans 17
Status epilepticus 10, 16, 18, 27, 41, 45, 88-90
    afebrile 12
    classification of 89
    convulsive 88, 91*fc*
    De novo 90
    epidemiology of 89
    etiology of 90*b*
    evaluation of 97*fc*
    febrile 9, 10, 14
    first-line antiepileptic drugs in 92*t*
    management of 90
    medical management of 90
    new onset refractory 90
    nonconvulsive 18, 88, 91*fc*, 96
    refractory 93
    second-line antiepileptic drugs in 92*t*
Stereotactic techniques 132
Steroids, high-dose 37
Stevens-Johnson syndrome 102
Stiripentol 72
Stokes-Adams syndrome 55
Stroke 56, 89, 90, 111
    like episodes 70
Supportive therapy 141
Surgically remediable syndromes 129
Syncope 17, 18, 30, 43, 54, 55, 55*t*
    common types of 55*b*
    convulsive 30
Systemic lupus erythematosus 32

T

Tachyarrhythmia 55
Taenia solium 34, 144
Teratogenesis, cognitive 50
Testis, undescended 49
Tetracyclic antidepressants, use of 61
Theophylline 43
Thiazides 43
Thrombocytopenia 92, 102
    transient 92
Thyroiditis, autoimmune 37
Thyrotoxicosis 41
Tiagabine 101
Tics 17
Todd's paresis 9
Tonic spasms 18
Tonic upward gaze, benign paroxysmal 17
Tonic-clonic seizure 18
    generalized 11, 18, 31, 44, 49, 110, 116
Topiramate 33, 51, 92, 100-102, 104, 125, 126
TORCH infections, congenital 111
Toxoplasmosis 36
Tramadol 32
Transcranial magnetic stimulation 93
Trauma 111
Tremor 102

Tricyclic antidepressants, use of 61
Tuberculoma, right parietal 35*f*
Tuberculosis 32, 34
    granuloma 34
Tumors 32, 36, 111
    low-grade 36
Typhoid 54

U

Unverricht-Lundborg disease 69, 70
Upper respiratory infection 8
Uremia 42
Urinary ketones 73
Urinary tract infection 8, 42

V

Vagal nerve stimulation 28, 127, 133
Valproate 12, 13, 33, 92, 100, 101, 105
Valproic acid 43, 44, 102
Vasculitis 32
Vasovagal syncope 30, 41
Venereal Disease Research Laboratory 38
Venlafaxine 61
Ventricular septal defect 49
Vertigo 92, 102
Video electroencephalography 85, 127
Vigabatrin 101, 104
Viral infections 8
Visual agnosia 64
Vitamin
    B_{12} 8
    D supplements 44

W

Weight
    gain 102
    loss 102
West's syndrome 80, 104
Wilder Graves Penfield 4
William Gordon Lennox 3
William Richard Gowers 3
Women with epilepsy 48
Women, epilepsy and pregnancy 48
World Health Organization 5

X

X-linked disorders 70

Y

Yoga, role of 151

Z

Zinc 8
Zonisamide 3, 102, 105, 125, 126

EU GSPR Authorised Reprsentative
Logos Europe, 9 rue Nicolas Poussin
1700, La Rochelle, France
Phone: +33 (0) 6 67 93 73 78
E-mail: contact@logoseurope.eu

www.ingramcontent.com/pod-product-compliance
Ingram Content Group UK Ltd.
Pitfield, Milton Keynes, MK11 3LW, UK
UKHW050428150426
5217IPUK00019B/1292